DIVORCE AS A
DEVELOPMENTAL PROCESS

Judith H. Gold, M.D., F.R.C.P.(C)
Series Editor

DIVORCE AS A
DEVELOPMENTAL PROCESS

Edited by

JUDITH H. GOLD, M.D., F.R.C.P.(C)

American
Psychiatric
Press, Inc.   1400 K Street, N.W.
Washington, DC 20005

Copyright © 1988 American Psychiatric Press, Inc.
All Rights Reserved
91 90 89 88 4 3 2 1

Manufactured in the U.S.A.

The paper used in this publication meets the minimum requirements of American National Standard for Information Sciences—Permanence of Paper for Printed Library Materials ANSI Z39.48-1984.   ∞

Library of Congress Cataloging-in-Publication Data

Divorce as a developmental process/edited by Judith H. Gold.
      p.   cm.—(Clinical insights)
  Includes bibliographies.
  ISBN 0-88048-146-3
  1. Divorce therapy. 2. Divorce—Psychological aspects.
3. Developmental psychology. 4. Adjustment
(Psychology)   I. Gold, Judith H., 1941– . II. Series.
  [DNLM: 1. Adaptation, Psychological. 2. Counseling.
  3. Divorce. 4. Social Adjustment.   WM55 D6185]
RC488.6.D56   1988
616.89—dc 19
DNLM/DLC   87-33685
for Library of Congress   CIP

Contents

Contributors

Elissa P. Benedek, M.D.
Clinical Professor of Psychiatry,
University of Michigan Medical Center
Director, Research Training Center for Forensic Psychiatry,
Ann Arbor, Michigan

Leah J. Dickstein, M.D.
Associate Professor,
Department of Psychiatry and Behavioral Sciences,
University of Louisville,
Louisville, Kentucky

Edgar Gold, L.L.B., Ph.D.
Professor,
Faculty of Law,
Dalhousie University, Halifax, Nova Scotia

Judith H. Gold, M.D., F.R.C.P.(C)
Halifax, Nova Scotia

Martha Kirkpatrick, M.D.
Associate Clinical Professor,
School of Medicine,
University of California at Los Angeles

Michael F. Myers, M.D., F.R.C.P.(C)
Clinical Professor,
Department of Psychiatry,
University of British Columbia;
Department of Psychiatry,
Shaughnessy Hospital, Vancouver

Carol C. Nadelson, M.D.
Professor and Vice Chairman,
Department of Psychiatry,
Tufts University School of Medicine;
Director of Training and Education,
Department of Psychiatry,
Tufts-New England Medical Center Hospitals,
Boston, Massachusetts

R. James Williams, L.L.B., M.S.W., B.Sc.
Judge of the Family Court of Nova Scotia;
Lecturer, Dalhousie University,
Halifax, Nova Scotia

Introduction
to the Clinical Insights Series

*T*he Clinical Insights Series provides mental health–psychiatric clinicians with the most current information on a variety of topics of interest to them. These monographs are factual, up to date, and focused on areas of importance in daily professional interactions, whether in the private office, the outpatient clinic, or the inpatient unit. They are written for clinicians working in psychiatry and in other mental health professions.

Each year a number of monographs will be published dealing with all aspects of clinical practice. In addition, from time to time, a monograph may be revised and updated. Thus the Series will provide quick access to relevant and important areas of psychiatric practice. Some titles in the Series will be authored by a single expert; others will be edited by such an expert, who also will draw together other knowledgeable authors to produce a comprehensive overview of a topic.

Some of the monographs in the Clinical Insights Series will have their foundation in presentations at the annual meetings of the American Psychiatric Association. All will contain the most recent information on the subjects discussed. Within these compact volumes, theoretical and scientific data will be applied to clinical situations and case illustrations will be included, all with the practitioner in mind.

The topic of divorce is an appropriate one for a book in the Clinical Insights Series. As you will read in the following chapters, divorce is a very frequent occurrence in North American families and affects many thousands of adults and children annually. Divorce is one of the most stressful of life events and adversely influences the mental health and daily functioning of those involved in the process. This monograph reviews the literature on these effects of divorce but focuses mainly on the therapeutic intervention, in order to demonstrate to the clinician that marital dissolution can become a catalyst for the individual's subsequent psychosocial growth and development.

Judith H. Gold, M.D., F.R.C.P.(C)
Series Editor,
Clinical Insights Series

Introduction

In psychiatry's continuing attempt to comprehend the behavior of people, individuals are viewed not only in isolation but also in terms of their relationships and place within their family, society, and culture. They are examined by life stage, intellectual and emotional development, and capacity for intimacy. Further, their interpersonal ties are dissected as to quality and depth of interchange, dependency, trust, and age and stage appropriateness. Nowhere is this multiple approach more necessary than when dealing with a disintegrating marriage and the consequences of that disintegration upon the persons involved, whether the partners, their children, parents, or friends. Divorce can be examined as a part of the development of a person psychologically and socially. It can also be examined as a catalyst itself to the personal development of an individual.

This book is written from the perspective of divorce as a catalyst, to illustrate and discuss how such a life event, which is usually so destructive and traumatic, can eventually result in positive growth for the individual. This further personal development indeed may not have occurred if the marriage had remained intact, and its evolution may be predicated in some cases only by psychotherapy and in others by the coping skills engendered by the divorce itself. Unfortunately, those persons who do not go on from marital dissolution to increased self-awareness and maturation may later again make a choice of a partner based on familiar repetitive needs with the same disastrous consequences.

The focus of this book is clinical and therapeutic, presenting the most recent knowledge of the effects of divorce at different stages of life and upon men and women. Although it is not a comprehensive look at all age groups and situations, the topics have been chosen to illustrate the most common and generalized reactions to divorce and its aftereffects on children, men, and women.

In Chapter 1, Leah Dickstein, M.D., writes about the psychosocial effects of personal divorce on young adults. She looks at the reasons why they divorce, especially in light of gender roles and cultural expectations for men and women. She describes the pressures exerted upon young people by the current social emphasis on material success and by narcissistic preoccupations. At the same time they strive to fulfill the new personal and social roles that have been outlined by changes in expectations of men and women in middle-class society, often without role models or an understanding of their own needs, assets, and abilities. The outcomes of divorce for these individuals, in terms of their future choices for themselves and of a new partner, are examined.

The divorce of a young couple also has effects upon their parents and the relationship between the divorced individuals and their parents. Dr. Dickstein views these relationships from the perspective of the adjustment during the divorce process itself.

In Chapter 2, Edgar Gold, L.L.B., Ph.D., and I discuss the belittling process, exploring the personal effects that today's changes in social and gender roles have on men and women within their marriage at all age levels. The belittling may begin as an attempt to regain or maintain a familiar balance in the relationship, as one partner struggles to keep an uncomfortable evolution from occurring. How this then affects personal development after divorce is important as both individuals struggle to restructure their lives and functioning.

Michael Myers, M.D., F.R.C.P.(C), provides a general discussion of the psychotherapeutic treatment of divorcing men in Chapter 3. He does not distinguish by age group or stage of personal development but looks globally at the common factors all men share, whether fathers or not. He examines the effect divorce has on the intrapsychic development of the man and upon his social functioning, while discussing the dynamics governing the man's behavior toward his former spouse, and perhaps children, and toward a therapist. Further, Dr. Myers points out countertransference issues important in treatment as well as in the training of young therapists.

In Chapter 4, Martha Kirkpatrick, M.D., provides more information on the societal changes that have led to the increased divorce rate in the last half of this century. The focus in this chapter, on women in their 40s and 50s, who are most vulnerable to the consequences of divorce, will help the clinician to appreciate the socioeconomic predicaments of these women, as well as their unique position between two social roles within a social evolution. Raised in a world that expected them to be wives and mothers, once divorced in middle age, many women suddenly find they are expected to become wage earners and be self-supporting. This is another example of the personal development necessitated by divorce and required for survival.

Little has been written about sexual behavior after divorce, especially from the perspective of its place within the developmental process after divorce. Dr. Myers describes some reactions in men, and Carol Nadelson, M.D., and I look at women's sexual interactions in Chapter 5. The focus here is on the effect of divorce upon the ability to trust and to be intimate with another.

Postdivorce development of children and adolescents is discussed by Elissa Benedek, M.D., in Chapter 6. Dr. Benedek reviews the extensive literature on the severe psychological stress placed upon the children of divorce and the consequences for their personal development and subsequent ability to be intimate and choose partners. Dr. Benedek emphasizes the need for a child to continue to have loving, consistent relationships with both parents throughout the growing years and into young adulthood.

Judge James Williams, L.L.B., M.S.W., B.S., follows then with his perspectives as a family law practitioner and now judge in a family court, by pointing out that legal training does not prepare a lawyer to be a counsellor. In Chapter 7 he stresses that lawyers may not be capable of considering the psychological and social developmental impact of the marital disintegration and of the divorce process. However, this is necessary in order to provide a client with effective advice and legal services. He describes the psychological stages of divorce a lawyer should consider, as well as the need to properly assess what is best for any children involved.

The final chapter deals with the psychotherapeutic treatment of a divorcing person, again from the viewpoint of resultant developmental growth. I discuss the original needs brought to a marriage, including the differing growth of the capacity for intimacy between men and women, and how these affect the course of the marriage—as well as the divorce. I describe the stages of the divorce process and how therapists must consider these while utilizing the practical aspects of the legal divorce to evoke personal growth and change.

The importance of recognition by the therapist of the divorcing person's place in his or her life cycle, culture, and society is emphasized throughout this monograph. It is essential if therapeutic change is to be effective. For the men, women, and children involved, divorce, so common today—indeed so familiar, can be used to catalyze constructive individual psychological development.

Throughout the book, case examples are provided to illustrate the themes of each chapter and the points made. Thus the book should be useful to clinicians who have to deal with individuals and families suffering from the repercussions of divorce.

This monograph has its origins in a symposium on divorce presented by some of the authors at the annual meeting of the American Psychiatric Association in Washington, D.C., in 1986. However, all of the chapters have been written especially for this publication and do not appear elsewhere.

Divorce is not widely discussed in the psychiatric literature, as readers will note when examining the references for each chapter. However, there is a wide nonpsychiatric literature dealing with various aspects of family therapy and with divorce; of especial interest is the *Journal of Divorce*. Despite the lack of psychiatric literature on the topic, many psychiatric patients are exposed to divorce or to its effects because of the frequency of divorce at this time in North America. This experience is a profound one for the person and the family, and it is hoped that this monograph will illuminate the process for the clinician's greater understanding.

Judith H. Gold, M.D., F.R.C.P.(C)

Chapter 1

The Psychosocial Effects of Personal Divorce on Young Adults

LEAH J. DICKSTEIN, M.D.

Chapter 1

The Psychosocial Effects of Personal Divorce on Young Adults

*T*oday's young adults experienced little of the early effects of the second women's movement in the United States, which began its focus on equality in 1963, following publication of Betty Friedan's classic book, *The Feminine Mystique*, and her leadership in helping to organize the National Organization for Women in 1966. Only a minority of young mothers in the early 1960s were able to choose to personalize the issues and effect changes for themselves and their families (1). This select group was drawn largely from the college-educated white women volunteers who had struggled so vigorously and so naturally for others' benefit in the civil rights crusade of the 1950s.

Like so many generations before them, these women's sex role socialization was different from that of the men. Their overriding directive had been something like the following: "BE helpful, polite, and attractive to others first, and consequently you will be valued and liked by them and therefore can find yourself worthy." The expectations for the men were different: "DO what it takes to succeed and be proud of yourself. Compete and win for yourself; others will be pleased, and, of course, you will also be responsible for, protect, and love your family."

For the first time in decades, perhaps in all history, countless women in the 1960s thought and felt that doing something for themselves was legitimate. These were not the women who were forced to work out of economic necessity. The earliest issues that these women faced included opportunities for work and careers outside the home even if they had children, higher education, and entry into the male-dominated professions or into nontraditional jobs.

Along with deciding to and actually entering the work force, these women hesitatingly attempted to renegotiate primary personal responsibilities for home, husband, and children with their husbands. The husbands in turn reacted with confusion at best and commonly with anger, because they had never expected this turn of events in their lives. These women, and most women and many men since the early 1960s, understand why women assign greater importance to equality and personal independence than men do. Clearly their sex role socialization and life experiences have shown women that men's values are equated with "all people" and "our society" while for the most part women's values have not been recognized or considered.

As children born in the late 1950s, when Simone de Beauvoir's book, *The Second Sex*, had already crossed the Atlantic from France, today's young adults were reared in traditional sociocultural environments. These children also counted on mothers, but not fathers, to be at home and available on a full-time basis to meet their school, extra-curricular, and leisure time needs and desires. They also expected their mothers to keep the home and all its contents presentable in a loving and giving manner without asking the children to assume very many responsibilities. The children knew that their fathers, the wage earners, naturally made most family decisions. Their primary caregivers, nuclear and extended families, and preschool women teachers were perhaps beginning to be aware of possible gender role issues through the media, but they had not usually allowed themselves to become personally involved or directly affected by these new proposals (2).

Furthermore, although the first men's movement for equality in the United States ensued in the early 1970s, itself called the Decade of Choice, fewer repercussions were felt from this movement and by smaller numbers of adults. As the leaders of the women's movement had previously been involved in the civil rights movement, many of the small handful of men involved in the men's movement had earlier been involved in and learned from the women's movement. These men were emotionally healthy enough to admit that women ought to be allowed choices in all areas of their lives and that they themselves needed and wanted more work and personal options as well as more direct recognition, expression, and sharing of feelings with their significant others, their friends, and, if they were parents, their children. Generally speaking, the life-styles of adults who were affected neither by the men's movement nor the women's movement of the 1960s were observed by the young adults of today as the latter experienced increasing gender role pressures and biologic stages of adolescence in the 1970s.

Thus we should be neither surprised nor shocked that the divorce rate among young adults in the late 1980s is high and that divorce is more culturally acceptable, despite the fact that the pertinent and multifaceted psychosocial factors implicated in these divorces have been part of the mental health literature for some time: choices in education, work sought to support oneself and/or one's family, personal choices of whether or not to be involved in a significant adult emotional relationship (whether heterosexual, homosexual, or bisexual), whether to have biologic children or to adopt someone else's, and all of the repercussions these choices imply. If one chose marriage, then when? If one chose to have children, then when? If both partners work outside the home, then whose work is deemed more important when crises (for example, health or job opportunities) arise?

These young people developed in a culture that emphasized the importance of achievement, upward mobility, the buying power of the successful, and the expected pattern of re-

5

placing what was out of style when something better came on the market rather than keeping an article until it was very old and irreparable (planned obsolescence). For example, new cars, new clothing, new homes, hair styles, capped teeth, breast implants, the stock market—all quick fixes easily obtained without much waiting, planning, and hard work—were based on the value "why not care and do for myself?": The Me Generation. From one standpoint, marriage might be viewed as another aspect of one's somewhat narcissistic life that can be changed easily (3).

For young adults who belonged to racial, religious, and ethnic minorities, choices were more limited. Their frustrations were more widespread and more nearly devastating.

In fact, many of these young adults may have intellectually grasped the new psychological concepts as they grew up but did not truly understand, nor internalize, the changing roles for women and men and their consequent changing lifestyles. This lack of true insight, which might have precipitated behavior change, appeared in these young adults because they were so immersed in options that differed from their parents' and grandparents' alternatives. They were without adult role models who were living out, rather than merely espousing, the changing standards. These young adults could "talk a good game" with their peers, and even significant others, until they married and reality struck. They have had to learn about the new psychology of women and men through personal trauma. Those who have been healthy enough have recognized their problems and needs and made consequent efforts in psychotherapy.

Method

I reviewed 40 case histories, selected at random from my clinical experiences over the past 12 years with a university population. I shall highlight common, major, relevant psychosocial factors among these divorced young adults and include a number of vignettes to illustrate their major interactional patterns.

Briefly, though the psychosocial effects of a young adult's divorce are not necessarily all negative or chronic, many are devastating: loss of affection and emotional bonding; loss of the spouse role and of a significant other who was trusted and depended upon on many levels, both consciously and unconsciously; and finally, economic hardship. Clearly present are acute personal symptoms of high stress, anxiety, depression, guilt, helplessness, anger, envy, shame, humiliation, despair, suicidal ideation, failure, conversion symptoms, and sexual disorders—very painful emotions and conditions.

The positive psychosocial effects are often overlooked, but as ways to maintain and build self-esteem in a tumultuous period, they should be recognized and explored. The positive outgrowths may be initial relief that a decision was made and tension decreased; recognition of and responsibility for an error in partner choice; realization of the existence of poor or no effective communication skills; an end to misinterpreting and making incorrect assumptions in the relationship; improper work choice or goal, or lack of either; disagreement in matters relating to contraception, abortion, and child rearing; and disagreement in dealing with parents, ex-spouses, and children. In addition, competition outside the home in the work arena and now at home for love, attention, and responsibilities was a major, though rarely admitted issue, for everyone concerned in the sample I examined.

Importantly, the young adults, having divorced and been in psychotherapy, can then realize what future choices they want and how they will change their most basic communication methods.

Factors Pertaining Primarily to the Men

The age range was 23 to 32 among the 20 men. They were all Caucasian and either Catholic or Protestant. Half were left by their wives. Most of the wives worked outside the home, several as professionals, others in white-collar jobs. The majority of the wives were college graduates, usually only a year or two younger than their husbands. The couples had married in their very early 20s, and a common complaint was that voiced by one wife to her husband as "I haven't had fun or experienced enough of life and dated too little. You barely take an interest in me; we don't communicate well on verbal, emotional, or sexual levels. We also don't spend emotionally intimate, good times together, and I've decided I don't want to wait for us to reach better times!" This woman's expression of frustration and disappointment echoed what Lillian Rubin in 1983 described in men's and women's relationships as "intimate strangers, i.e., those who struggle to reconcile men's desire for separation and women's desire for union" (4). Now in their mid to late 20s, these women felt that "time was of the essence," and they did not want to lose more than the few years they had already invested in their marriages.

A significant number of the wives admitted that social standing and economic comfort acquired through their husbands' employment was not worth the personal sacrifices of self-actualization. At one time, money had been important as they emerged into adulthood, yet now it needed to be inserted into their hierarchy of values in its proper place.

Furthermore, although only four had children, being a parent was not seen as a strong dissuading factor against divorce.

Most of the men came seeking therapy late in the dissolution of the marriage. They were stereotypically socialized to refrain from showing and sharing emotions and asking for help. In this instance, they paid a high price for being burdened with this negative trait.

The women felt that since their marriages, they had matured, gained self-confidence, and modified and changed their life goals, priorities, and coping strategies. In some instances they cited development of personal life goals where previously none had existed. To the contrary, they felt their husbands had remained unchanged personally and were as traditional in life outlook and behavior as their own fathers and mothers.

In 20 percent of the reviewed divorces, the wives were brought to therapy, initially because they were depressed, by the men who were too busy in school to come but felt fine themselves. Only after the wives' evaluations were the husbands invited to a joint session; they then entered therapy, and the complete picture of marital dissolution became apparent.

In three instances, young men sought individual therapy to gain advice about short-term dyadic therapy with the fore-warning that they would then withdraw and their wives would have therapists when the men sought divorce. The men's guilt was obvious, and they were aware of it.

In other cases, after being confronted with the divorce news, the rejected men felt devastated. Consequently, they were willing to "do anything to make the marriage work," including looking at and modifying their values about personal power, responsibility, and choice for each spouse; acknowledging their differing and changing roles; entering couple therapy; and promising to help more at home and pay more attention to their wives' needs and interests. With a perceived loss of control over their lives, the men felt they were forfeiting their identity and therefore felt disoriented, confused, and empty.

Women had experienced this identity loss for all of history, having been socialized to be comfortable in being *Mrs.* Bob Jones (and to some extent they still do, witness *Mrs.* Mary Smith-Jones). The men and women who entered therapy learned at some point that they needed better skills to develop first a healthy personal identity and, second, a constructive, intimate relationship.

Sellner's description parallels the reactions of this male cohort: Men "are probably devastated the most when relationships break up. Women experience what you would call heartbreak. Men experience a kind of breaking of the spirit. It's often harder for them to carry on, and they often don't understand the split" (5). In one instance, a young man developed conversion symptoms and was hospitalized on the psychiatric unit for 10 days.

Although a few therapy sessions took place in which the wife's complaints were aired and discussed and options to correct them were enumerated, usually the wives eventually followed through with the divorce.

The men did, in fact, attempt to modify their behavior in a number of important and specific ways. For example, they made genuine efforts to spend more time with their wives by cutting back on studying time and on other out-of-the-home commitments, including less time "out with the boys for sports or a beer." They suggested going out to dinner, dancing, or attending a movie or concert. They offered sports time with their wives rather than with their male friends, despite the "lack of real competition." They actually assumed a more active role with housekeeping chores. They were more demonstrative emotionally, both verbally and physically.

What the men in the present sample often felt after making these changes can be expressed by Freud's comment in a letter to a female colleague decades ago: "What do women want? They will have to figure it out for themselves" (6). The women often stated that "love was not enough," and they would now seek genuine friendship, emotional intimacy, and personal equality in future relationships. These women often acknowledged that they had married in good faith, that is, expecting their commitment "to be forever" like their parents' marriages, although at the same time they felt they were more aware than their mothers were of the respective roles of husband and wife. However, after a while, they realized that the personal cost of maintaining the relationship for others' approval, namely, husbands, parents, and in-laws, would be too high. Consequently these young women often found themselves without family support, for early on their shocked parents often sided with their sons-in-law.

For these women, socialized to be more dependent and acquiescent than their brothers, going against their parents' and husband's wishes for the marriage to remain intact was often a first major step toward mature separation and individuation. The adjustment was not easy. Often the women had no recognizable support system until they began verbalizing more to others at work and at school, started group or individual therapy, or joined informal consciousness-raising groups. While these new contacts were being made, these young women cared for themselves, often for the first time in their lives, and were unsure and lonely at times, but with hesitant steps plodded on. Supported and strengthened primarily by their own new convictions, they progressed, building on each small success and overcoming mistakes when they faltered. Despite the higher levels of jobs and the increased number of professions open to women, since most young women earn 64 cents to the men's dollar, they also experienced economic pressures. The current feminization of poverty is serious and widespread.

The rejected young men often displayed heretofore unrecognized passivity and major dependency needs, what I refer to as "the white knight syndrome" (7). In this syndrome, men appear to be very independent and self-sufficient at work, deny their emotions, act as competent leaders in their personal relationships, and also care for their significant woman, who assumes a wife's traditional dependent role. On an unconscious level, these men often expected their young wives to care for them as their mothers had, although when questioned they at first denied it. For most men, turning to male friends was difficult and awkward. They were unused to sharing failures, helplessness, and tears with other men. For the women, a support system was much easier to find and more valuable.

Chemical dependence was not an issue for these men or for their spouses. The men placed a high premium on work and personal success. Several had changed careers and were able to accomplish the switch because their wives, as expected, without complaint or resistance and with seeming pleasure, were their financial mainstays. The majority divorced during graduate and professional training, so their wives may have supported them financially through undergraduate as well as part of their postgraduate training. Other men expressed their own ambivalence about their marriages. A number of them evidenced obsessive–compulsive features, could not deal with anger directly on a verbal basis, and had unfinished childhood developmental issues to resolve, including incomplete separation and individuation.

Several of the men had strong religious convictions that their wives later stated often adversely affected their sexual and marital relationships. These particular men belonged to fundamentalist sects and adhered to prescribed sexual practices, which were unlike the increased liberties, openness, and enjoyment that most youth touted in the 1970s and 1980s regarding sexual practices. Unknowingly, these men had thought their religion was a common marital bond. They believed the structure offered by their church gave the women the same security that they as men felt. Raised by conservative parents with whom they had had little or no discussion about sex, they then had either superficial or no conversation about sexual practices and preferences with their wives. Church directives to the women about sex as a duty to the husband and to the couple to bear children provided relief from risk taking in sharing sexually for mutual pleasure.

Case Example 1

John was 26 years old and had been married to Mary for four years. They had met at a church social, dated for three years, and continued to live at home until they graduated from college and married. Each had had part-time jobs to help with expenses while parents paid for tuition. For both, the relationship was their first on a long-term basis.

After their marriage, Mary worked as a teacher and was compliant in all the couple's mutual decisions. John had changed careers from teaching to medicine, spent hours in class and studied even more than most of his classmates.

They attended church regularly and saved their money for home purchases he wanted, such as the compact discs and state-of-the-art stereo and camera equipment. They rarely did anything for fun in a spontaneous or even planned way, communicated only superficially, and shared sexually about once every week or two at her suggestion. Neither expressed any anger, disappointment, or joy about their relationship. In the year before she left the marriage, Mary spent more time in social relationships with female co-workers and began night classes toward an advanced degree. She had not discussed returning to school with John to any extent. She had simply signed up, she said, to keep busy, and he replied with "sure" and asked no further questions.

John had thought they were happy, so he concentrated his thoughts and energy on his work and his future, which he thought included Mary. In a state of shock, he cried for two weeks straight after Mary left home. He turned for solace, support, and answers to his parents, in-laws, friends—anyone—just so he wouldn't be alone. He felt unable to function and could not sleep, study, or eat; he felt humiliated, guilty, and abandoned and only occasionally angry enough to want revenge.

After several couple therapy sessions, Mary filed for divorce, and they shared a lawyer to save money in this uncontested action. John gave her anything she wanted from their property in the hope she would change her mind. He was aghast that she could think of giving up their future and her secure role as a physician's wife for the opportunities to meet more people, get her own further education, perhaps change jobs or careers, allow herself to enjoy frivolous activities, and fantasize about seeking a different kind of heterosexual relationship! As he thought back to their three-year courtship, he realized they had not done any of the things Mary now wanted. During what he now recognized as those superficially pleasant years, he had assumed a great deal, especially that she simply wanted everything he did and would happily comply with his long-standing personal plans.

In individual sessions, and later all-male group therapy, John slowly began to recognize the very real problems in their relationship: their lack of communication on many levels; his lack of visible interest in her as a separate person; and, of paramount importance, his inadequate appreciation of her individual needs, thoughts, and interests. With concerted effort, he admitted his real but unrecognized emotional and personal dependency upon his wife and his parents. He courageously remained in therapy and faced these issues and, fortunately for him, did not immediately find another woman to take Mary's place, as many other men too often do.

For the men who divorced their wives, the reasons were similar to those of the wives who initiated divorce proceedings. These men stated they felt *they* had changed, that is, had new interests, values, and goals, but that their wives had not grown personally. Whether the wives worked outside the home in jobs or careers or were full-time housewives caring for children seemingly made no difference. These men felt bored, distant, and dissatisfied in their marital relationships.

Two divorced their mentally ill wives after psychiatric treatment did not seem to be resolving the problems. One divorced because, despite couple and individual therapy, the husband was not satisfied with the frequency of their sexual contact, insisting, "I can't live this way."

Several also admitted that they were dissatisfied with themselves and needed to "find themselves" but wanted to do it alone, apart from the marriage. For some this was the case even though they had lived independently or with male peers through college prior to meeting their future wives. A few had lived with these women for up to three years before they married.

There was a striking lack of willingness to struggle and grow together, even at different rates and in some different directions that they could still share and even if they still voiced love for their partners, which several did. The men uniformly said they didn't realize the real implications of changing roles, choices, and equality for women and men. Before the crisis of their divorce, they had not been forced to confront these new options, nor the concomitant stressful yet rewarding opportunities for personal growth and changing lifestyles.

For the most part, the men observed that their parents enjoyed, tolerated, or did not expect different lifestyles from the inception of their marriage to the present time, except for increasing economic security. Their mothers were definitely not feminists but were instead rather conservative. Without higher education, technical skills, or recent work experience, these mothers had, or assumed they had, fewer options to be on their own, so they had not ever seriously contemplated divorce as a viable option.

Factors Pertaining Primarily to the Women

Among the 20 women, the age range was 24 to 35. They were all Caucasian and either Catholic or Protestant. All the women initially verbalized grateful relief once they had made the decision to divorce. As a group, they willingly sought therapy sooner than the men, which is characteristic of women in general. Among them, two of the husbands had developed chemical addictions, including alcohol and narcotics. One of the two, Jerry, became violent during the last few years of the marriage and threatened and abused his wife Sally by blackening her eyes, beating her, threatening to shoot her, taking away her car keys and money, and breaking into their house while they were temporarily separated. She feared for her life and on several occasions called the police. Jerry refused professional help, blaming all his problems on Sally's being in school. At one point he did see a psychiatrist, who concurred with the husband, stating if Sally would simply stay home, all of Jerry's problems would vanish!

The second husband was supportive of his wife's career but stole drugs, was arrested repeatedly, accepted psychiatric hospitalization, and upon discharge after two months, returned to school only to resume drug theft and abuse.

Both women attempted to get psychiatric help for their husbands; they were willing to enter dyadic therapy and remained in the marriage until relapses became chronic. The women then chose not to continue what they saw as a destructive and hopeless marriage.

In another case, Beth divorced because her husband confessed to having an affair with another woman but did not evidence much appropriate, or at least expected, remorse. Paula divorced because she felt rejected by her husband, who was always disinterested in sexual relations, and was tired of insisting upon it and succeeding once or twice a year. She also felt rejected because he was neither financially nor emotionally supportive of her career change. To be completely honest, Paula had to admit that she had shied away from sharing with him during their courtship and live-in months and that since adolescence she had held a dream of becoming a lawyer.

Lack of support for the woman's changing role from traditional wife or wife and mother to working woman or student and wife and mother was common and a major cause for the woman to divorce.

Case Example 2

Nancy was the eldest of three children. Her father abused alcohol and her mother. Nancy watched helplessly, and her mother took the abuse until the father decided to leave the family permanently for his latest girlfriend. Nancy admitted she had married in the mid-1970s simply as the only way she felt comfortable to bear a child, which she wanted desperately. She then divorced after three years when she felt she and her husband, Robert, had nothing in common besides the child. He was rarely around to spend time with the child and in fact has become a better father since her second marriage to Ben. Now Robert actually pays attention to their son when he cares for him, asking what activities would please him, what he would like to eat, how he is doing in school, and about his friends.

Nancy, although wanting companionship and thinking she and Ben were compatible, divorced a second time after two years, feeling this second husband was too strict with her child, too compulsive about their home, and too involved with his mother.

Three women divorced because their husbands refused to help with child care after the birth of their children, although the men had made this commitment before the mutually planned pregnancy occurred. These women worked or were in school. At first they attempted "to do it all," meeting their responsibilities as superwomen, mothers, and traditional wives in addition to career and professional responsibilities. Finally, in anger, irritation, and frustration, they sought a divorce when reasoning did not persuade their husbands to pitch in and desist from the latter's resentment. Along the way, the women realized insightfully and wisely that "superwoman" was a myth.

Role strain, that is, societal permission to pursue goals without community support agencies or arrangements to do so, has consistently affected women more than it has men, although this important factor is increasingly having impact on men.

Several women divorced after realizing they simply no longer loved their husbands. Two admitted to marrying at a young age to escape intolerable home situations, especially when chronic parental disharmony or divorce, parental alcoholism, or mental illness predominated.

Case Example 3

Josie divorced Eric because or in spite of the fact that he loved her and was supportive of her career. The elder of two children, she had spent her high school years caring for her mother, who chronically threatened suicide. Her father would alternately tell her to care for her mother and then, after drinking heavily, would menace his wife with a shotgun. Her father trusted no one when he was sober, and Josie felt safe only when she was protecting her parents, running the house, and parenting her brother.

Her parents finally divorced during her junior year in college, but she continued, even at a distance, to respond to their crises because both insisted therapy was useless.

After several unrewarding relationships with destructive men, she met Eric and married him although she knew she did not love him. He was as caring to her as she had been to her family, and although she appreciated his considerateness, she *could not tolerate* their relationship. A year after the divorce, she entered individual therapy, followed by an all-women's therapy group to begin her struggle with these issues.

Some women said they married the first man who asked and of whom their parents approved, finally conceding their own unresolved dependency.

One discovered her bisexuality during her marriage and sought a single lifestyle in order to pursue her personal and professional identity and development.

In therapy, a number of the women, often the eldest sibling, observed that their difficult husbands strikingly resembled the difficult fathers or mothers they thought they had separated from when they left home and married.

Those young women who divorced because they felt a lack of communication and emotional and sexual intimacy in their marriage did not choose to make the effort to seek conjoint therapy. Rarely did the couple who could communicate effectively divorce because they had "grown apart." In fact, they had discovered what they identified as more compatible partners.

Case Example 4

An interesting note is that among all of these 20 educated women, only 1 was divorced by her husband. Elizabeth was a 25-year-old junior medical student when she entered therapy with the chief complaint of "my marriage is falling apart; can you help?"

She and her 27-year-old engineer husband had met and married during undergraduate days. They had shared an interest in sports, and Elizabeth attended all his baseball games, assumed most of their household tasks, and gained admission to medical school. Dennis was quiet, very pleasant, overweight, and honest about his dislike of not knowing when Elizabeth would be home each night. He had accepted and tolerated her preclinical years, had been very cooperative with less time together, and did some of the shopping and cooking, and Elizabeth still attended his games.

Dennis took time from his job so they could come to therapy together regularly and talked about his feelings of abandonment and loneliness. She offered to withdraw from medical school. He said he could not let her do that and would try to adjust. His mother was a high-school-graduated, full-time homemaker who offered to cook all his meals if Elizabeth could not get home in time or at all. Elizabeth's mother was a teacher who, though proud of her daughter, did wish she would not work so hard and would begin a family.

After several months in therapy, they stopped coming, and one month later, a few weeks before graduation, Elizabeth came to say Dennis had filed for divorce. She seemed stronger in that a decision had been made and she was going to another city for her residency. She realized without much apparent anger that he simply needed and wanted an enormous amount of support, and as much as she offered, it was not enough.

Also important is the sharp contrast in initial reactions to imminent divorces for the two sexes. With the exception of Josie, these women gained insight and felt a new healthy sense of personal power to control their lives. The opposite effect usually occurred in the men when they confronted upheaval in their relationships. At first they felt an increasing powerlessness and consequently became very symptomatic. Several became suicidal and were hospitalized. They could only voice feelings that their ideal, special woman, their lover and helper in pursuit of their life's dream, had changed! This extreme rejection reaction is seen increasingly among men and less among women at university counseling centers and mental health services nationally.

The women did not enter new relationships as quickly as the men. Many, in fact, enjoyed their first-time experience of economic and personal self-sufficiency and independent living.

Case Example 5

Marie was 27 and had married at 20. She met Tom, now 29, while both were in college and was grateful to be asked, and relieved to avoid spinsterhood, when he proposed marriage. Their early years together were traditional. Tom worked and tried to get ahead in his job, while Marie also worked but focused more on the appearance of their home and wondered when they would start a family.

After several years, she started listening to other women at work and began reading magazines and books for women about career and employment opportunities of all kinds. She became energized and enthralled with the idea of fulfilling her childhood fantasy of becoming a lawyer, which her family had discouraged. Tom seemed surprised at her sudden desire to pursue professional education. He became quiet, though not outwardly angry, and withdrew emotionally and sexually. Marie entered law school and gradually became more assertive.

Now becoming emotionally closer to her classmates, she felt distanced from Tom at home. Their sexual relationship became nonexistent as she grew more assertive, and he withdrew to sleep. Tom refused to seek counseling when she suggested it, and after two years Marie filed for divorce.

After she moved out, they both experienced depression at first, and Marie harbored a great deal of guilt, but in therapy she worked through these issues. She realized in part she had married to avoid the risk of becoming an old maid, something her mother had harped on during Marie's teenage years. Marie also discovered that her father's well-meaning, overprotective attitude had instilled in her the feeling that she could but should never attempt to excel at anything, except managing her home, and especially in a predominant male occupation. She gradually gained insight into Tom's, her parents', and her own old and new attitudes and values about role changes and choices for women and men. As she began widening her social sphere and her functioning improved, she slowly adapted to an independent living situation, something she had never before experienced and in fact had thought she was incapable of handling.

Discussion

Evident in this small sample of divorced young adults is that psychosocial issues relating to the new psychology of women and men were important precipitating factors in the demise of their marriages. Unfortunately, these psychosocial issues went unrecognized early in the dissolution of the relationships.

Clearly, basic options for current adulthood must include changing roles and the possibility of new choices in roles, particularly for women in work outside the home and for men in personal relationships and responsibilities at home. New styles in relationships must include the unquestionable need for both partners to communicate verbally in a direct manner and on a continual basis, a situation that has not often existed in traditional marriages. Seidenberg's description of a traditional relationship consisting of one and one-half people, where the wife is the half who is compliant and quiet, will not suffice for most young women and men in relationships today (8).

Most of the young men, once they married, expected traditional wives no matter how they had related to these women before the ceremony. Indeed, most of the young women had similar expectations for themselves, whatever their educational level, professional accomplishments, or work responsibilities actually were at the time of marriage.

Conscious efforts by therapists must be directed toward encouraging young adults to risk resolving earlier developmental issues such as separation, individuation, self-understanding, identity, and acceptance before entering relationships. Otherwise, both participants can complicate matters by imitating unrecognized, destructive parental patterns. Furthermore, young women and men must develop comfort rather than feelings of discomfort and helplessness in verbalizing anger and other emotions in direct and constructive ways.

Therapists must always take into account the possibility of potential individual psychopathology in all initial evaluations of young adults in marital crisis. Personal mental or physical illness; unresolved issues related to gender identity or abandonment secondary to being adopted; the addicting disorders—alcohol, drug abuse, eating, and gambling; the phobic, anxiety, and the affective disorders; and the personality disorders must all be ruled out before the focus in therapy turns to sociocultural and psychosocial issues. Intellectualizing and denying problems in an age of nuclear family isolation, complicated dual work lifestyles, and economic and political uncertainty can often signal the death knell of a marriage that has only just begun.

Yet men are socialized to avoid asking for help, and most

adhere to this cultural guideline. Levinson, in *The Seasons of a Man's Life*, states that most men in their 20s are not ready to make an enduring inner commitment to wife and family and are not capable of a highly loving, sexually free, and emotionally intimate relationship. Rather, they are still separating from parents (9). We often overlook the cultural dogma that men take for granted their rights to independent action, while women may be more aware of the difficulties in reconciling the pull toward close attachments in their newly legitimized desire for individual development.

Increasingly, men who are divorcing seek sole or joint custody of their children. Although at the turn of this century men unquestionably gained responsibility for their children, this changed decades ago. In many instances, these young men want to be, and in fact are, as effective fathers to their children as their wives are mothers, and so they must be considered responsible and loving guardian parents.

Many may be able to acknowledge verbally that our age is one in which changing roles and a multitude of outside-the-home personal and professional options are numerous, especially for women. Yet young adults, reared in a traditional environment, find it difficult to actually understand and tolerate the emotional sacrifices, stresses, strains, *and* satisfactions they will experience if they actualize these new choices for themselves or support their partners in doing so. We do our young adults a disservice if we encourage them to make these new choices without helping them to develop the skills necessary to understand and deal with the personal as well as psychological and social costs involved.

Before they contemplate the possibility of a successful marriage, young adults must surmount the stages of basic trust and moderate separation–individuation. They must have in place communication skills about sex and work, sensitivity to another's needs, and awareness of personal strengths and weaknesses.

What is disconcerting about divorce as an option for young adults becomes understandable when we realize that their parent role-models waited for many more painful years to divorce at ages 40, 50, 60 or beyond. Instead, these parents may have lived lives of quiet or noisy desperation and unhappiness, and primarily the mothers may never have attempted to self-actualize in significant ways. Their children, our current young adults, observed their parents' unhappiness, yet too often unconsciously adopted the same ineffective methods of coping and communicating.

The effects of their parents' divorce upon young adults should not be overlooked or minimized. The parents' divorce may have occurred at any stage of the child's development from preschool to college and still be extremely traumatic for these young persons, who may not fully understand the parents' personal and marital dynamics that led to the divorce. For too many parents, embroiled in and saddened by their own emotions, do not share, and the apparently sophisticated adult children do not question.

Among the 40 cohorts, 25 percent experienced parental divorce and in consultation obviously still had unresolved feelings about it. They also felt responsible to be supportive to both parents, although they often expressed helplessness and anger in this role of parenting their parents.

Regardless of the socioeconomic status of the parents, alcohol abuse was a common occurrence among the older adults, although it did not always lead to divorce, particularly if the alcohol problem was the father's.

Notable is that seven of the men and six of the women had parents who divorced. Three of the men had fathers who abused alcohol. One woman had a father and a mother who abused alcohol. Two of the men came from an abusive family. One father in a rage burned all the family furniture in the front yard. Another father chronically psychologically and occasionally physically abused all three sons. Three of the women had mothers who were identified as mentally ill. A history of family violence in parents including spouse and child abuse and incest are commonly implicated in destroying young adults' potentially good marriages.

However, what is encouraging is that many of these young adults have postponed bearing children during the early years of their marriage and thus fewer "helpless others," that is, children, are secondarily affected. Rewarding, too, is the fact that an increasing number of young adults enter therapy, initially for crisis intervention but often continue on in psychodynamic therapy, gain insight, and later choose partners more wisely and interact with them in more sensitive ways.

Divorced young adults need support and guidance as they reenter the singles' world. The bar scene becomes distasteful in short order. Consequently, matchmaker style services of all types are proliferating, from actual matchmakers to video agencies, newspaper and magazine ads, bachelor auctions, and organized singles' groups. The latter are sometimes based on special interests such as reading, sports, and travel. Churches offer group counseling, universities provide continuing education courses, and media programs deal with the issues and problems confronting today's singles. The adults themselves, in mixed or same-sex groups, discuss money; housing; child rearing; loneliness; dating; sexual drives; new spouses, ex-in-laws, and family members; hobbies; and career plans.

The influence of all forms of the media, particularly television, cannot be glossed over. Young adults watch thousands of hours of fantasy, instant access, change, violence, and the "soaps." For many who live at a distance from scattered, extended families, the "soap families" become their own, and they rush home from school and work to watch "my favorite soap." TV's comedies, dramas, and series too often emphasize simplistic, superficial solutions. They permit extreme verbal and physical violence and abuse, allowing little or no creative answers to problems. Television addicts are spoon-fed explanations rather than being challenged to find independent ones based on individual effort.

Saturday morning cartoons added to unrealistic and stereotypic beliefs through direct and subliminal messages—men *do*, achieve, have fun, and win the girl; women *be*, always thin, young, sexy, and helpful to others.

Divorced young adults could also probably benefit from some cultural ritual to demarcate the divorce event aside from a lonely trip to the courthouse or lawyer's office to sign papers or receiving a registered letter in the mailbox. Informing co-workers, peers, and all levels of both families, and certainly the children, is presently haphazardly accomplished at best. Research into discarded divorce customs of orthodox religions or creation of new rites would serve a useful purpose.

Perhaps the divorce rate will decrease as psychosocial and sociocultural issues and the "new psychology of women and men" are confronted by younger children and adolescents at an earlier age and in a more meaningful way in incorporated core classes in our middle and high schools. The risk of not exposing these youngsters to these new concepts in a constructive manner at an appropriately early developmental stage is too costly!

Conclusion

Mental health professionals must first steep themselves in the literature of the new psychology of men and women, then admit to themselves their own feelings, limitations, and biases regarding these changes, which have been called the most powerful of this century. Therapists must become aware, as Adams has stated, that "sexist attitudes and behaviors on an individual level are socially sanctioned and reproduced, and political structures and hierarchies shape individual feelings, attitudes and behaviors" (10).

If therapists can be knowledgeable, ready, and available for the young adults who are emotionally healthy enough to seek therapy and risk personal growth and change, then stable, rewarding relationships can be a plausible part of their futures.

I am pleased to report that all 40 young adults in the present cohort group have progressed to more mature personal identities and life functioning and feel better about themselves. The majority have entered new, sound unions, willing and able to view marriage as an opportunity to allow both partners continued personal growth potential based on mutual trust. Finally, they feel competent to cope more constructively and happily in an intimate relationship that they expect to continue well into the 21st century.

References

1. Friedan B: The Feminine Mystique. New York, Dell, 1977
2. de Beauvoir S: The Second Sex: The Classic Manifesto of the Liberated Woman. New York, Alfred A. Knopf, 1952
3. Rice JK, Rice DG: Living Through Divorce: A Developmental Approach to Divorce Therapy. New York, Guilford Press, 1986
4. Rubin L: Intimate Strangers. New York, Harper & Row, 1983
5. Read J: Men are people too! The Men's Journal for Men and Women, Winter 1985/86, p. 9
6. Freeman L, Stearn H: Freud and women. New York, Frederick Unger, 1981
7. Dickstein LJ: Social change and dependency in university men: the white knight complex unresolved. Journal of College Student Psychotherapy 1:31-41, 1986
8. Seidenberg R: The possibilities for marriage between equals. Presented at a seminar on human development and developmental psychiatry: new psychology of women and men, Western New York Psychoanalytic Society Meeting, Syracuse, NY, June 12, 1976
9. Levinson DJ: The Seasons of a Man's Life. New York, Alfred A. Knopf, 1978
10. Adams D: Stages of antisexist awareness and change for men who batter. Presented at the annual meeting of the American Psychological Association, Toronto, 1985

Chapter 2

Belittling: Psychosocial and Legal Considerations

JUDITH H. GOLD, M.D., F.R.C.P.(C)
EDGAR GOLD, L.L.B., Ph.D.

Chapter 2

Belittling: Psychosocial and Legal Considerations

*T*he final decades of the 20th century, like the first, are full of battlefields. Armed conflicts and revolutions are occurring in Afghanistan, Nicaragua, Lebanon, the Basque region of Spain, near the China-Vietnam border, and in the Horn of Africa, to mention only the most current ones. Revolutions are also occurring within societies, cultures, and religions. This upheaval is felt in relationships between men and women, both in a broad societal context and within individual couples, as well as in legal and political changes, demands, and debates.

In some countries, such as those governed by the laws of Islam, religious beliefs have led to increased restrictions and formalizations of traditional roles. Women have had to resume fundamentally based positions within their families and society. Many have done so willingly and have persuaded or coerced their sisters to do the same. They maintain these rules even when outside their country and culture, as witnessed in every city or university town in North America. In other nations, the resurgence of fundamental Christianity and Judaism have gone hand in hand with a return to more structured roles for women. This includes strong emphasis on the woman's place as being within the home as wife and mother. Once again America is being crisscrossed by women campaigning fervently for the rights of women, defined either in terms of their wifely and maternal duties or in terms of their individual growth, development, and basic human freedoms. Woloch's interesting book, *Women and the American Experience*, analyzes this historical pattern of movement of women's place in American society (1).

In times of national wars women are often released from many traditional paths and permitted by society to tread along, and even open up, new avenues. However, once the male labor force experiences unemployment, the opportunities for women shrink, always justified and portrayed as being in the interest of the family and thus of the greater nation. Women then return home, and gradually changes evolve again, always with the encouragement and permission of a few supportive fathers and husbands and through the leadership of a few vocal and committed women. Over the years the role of the press in these changes has been substantial, indeed pivotal; it will be mentioned again later in this chapter.

While the position of North American women in society has been greatly governed by political and economic exigencies, the same trend can also be found in other countries. Today in some areas women are fighting guerrilla wars alongside men and dying alongside men. The sociopolitical revolts in the Philippines and in Nicaragua are examples of this, while in Europe, the Middle East, and Japan, terrorist brigades have long had women members and leaders. This is equality, too, to die or kill equally with men for a cause.

Meanwhile, in many countries, the demands for equal rights and freedoms for men and women escalate and de-escalate as if with the tides of the ocean. In this case the ocean is the prevailing stance of the greater society, influenced not by the moon and sun, but by the marketplace and the pressures of national and international politics. Since the 1970s in the Western world the majority of women work outside the home. However, most also work within the home. This multijob situation is not always by choice but may be dictated by economic necessity. This is not freedom to choose an occupation. For many decades women of the middle classes fought for the right to have an education and a job outside the family. Now many are allowed this not out of choice but because they need the income for their family or themselves. Poorer women, immigrant women, and non-white women have always had to work without choice.

For other women, jobs in the marketplace signify their entry into the larger society as individuals with abilities and useful skills. Although rarely paid wages equal to those men receive for the same or equivalent work, they feel free to use their training or innate skills in the work world. This freedom has evolved from the first pioneering attempts of women to receive an education. In North America this process lagged behind that of Great Britain and some other European countries. However, women's schools for higher education and colleges became established slowly and with great effort in America in the late 1800s (1, 2). Many women, thus educated, became teachers or missionaries. Historians and sociologists point out that at the turn of the century educated women often chose to remain single. As exemplified by Jane Addams, such single women had an enormous freedom in the use of their education, usually supported by other women in similar positions.

The Depression years saw a retreat of women back into their homes as laws were passed prohibiting the employment of a married women who might "take" a job from an unemployed father and husband. World War II with its vast drain on manpower again drew women out of their houses and into factories, offices, and hospitals. When the men returned the women went home. As Solomon writes, "Liberal education had made a real difference in women's lives, but their choices were still limited by personal inhibitions as well as public barriers" (2).

At the same time, girls were urged to develop their "femininity" and skills in order to become better wives and mothers. Magazines and movies portrayed women happy in these roles and giving up work for the sake of a happy home. However, by the early 1960s girls were again being encouraged to broaden their education, and the number of women doing so and continuing on in jobs grew. Solomon (2) relates this change to the government's attempt to rectify the gap between the United States and the Soviet "Sputnik" program. Once again women were told they could utilize their full abilities because it suited the national need!

But this time, through the 1960s and 1970s women not only studied and worked outside the home, they also began to demand more. Most also married and had children, thus encountering the dilemma of balancing all of their roles, like a juggler, often with a keenly critical audience. The audience was and is composed of their own ego ideals, superego regulations, and the expectations perceived and assumed of others. Friedan illustrated this in the 1960s in *The Feminine Mystique* and in the 1980s in *The Second Stage* (3, 4). These works eloquently illustrate the paths women took over the years and their current dilemmas.

Women are now free to work as well as to be wives and mothers. Frequently they have found they have three jobs, all full-time, squeezed into each day. The term "superwoman" became popular as women strove to do all these thoroughly and well. They felt guilty if they could not be super at it, and were exhausted from trying; a whole generation of women complained of chronic fatigue. Magazines proliferated in order to tell them how to do it, and household appliances grew numerous, varied, expensive, and convenient. The microwave oven seems to epitomize it all. The busy working woman can prepare a wonderful meal in minutes without changing from a business suit, or can reheat the food without spoiling it. And go on working to pay for the convenience!

Meanwhile arguments continue about women's equality. Laws are passed or defeated, courts rule and are overturned. In some states women are entitled to maternity leave and to regain the same job afterward. In others they are not. Some women support the drive for an Equal Rights Amendment in the United States; many do not. They cannot agree if education is for a woman's own purposes as a person or for the enhancement of her maternal and wifely roles. Many men are equally undecided. But, as already indicated, the majority of women are working, marrying, and are having children. Many delay motherhood until their careers seem established or until they feel financially stable. These women often face other quandaries, such as whether to return to their outside jobs, how to find adequate babysitters or daycare centers, and whether to work full- or part-time.

Thus while women are now free to make choices that were not available to them earlier in this century, that freedom has a considerable price attached. Part of that price is paid within a woman as she makes her choices, and another part may be paid by the marriage. Sometimes both go hand in hand, aided by the actions and choices of her mate. Accordingly, it is first necessary to look at the choice to marry before discussing what can happen within the marriage and, of course, when a marriage breaks up.

Marriage

Individuals marry for any one or a combination of reasons. Children grow up expecting to marry, whether their parents are together or not, especially in the large middle class of our society. Popular television shows perpetuate the vision of the happy family with a wise, somewhat comical father and a pretty, somewhat dependent mother. The mother is usually managing an outside job or has returned to study in order to obtain a rewarding position. The children are attractive stereotypes, and all problems are usually solved in each episode!

Such images must be very persuasive for young adolescents in the process of identity formation and individuation. Erikson taught us that from such identity develops the capacity to be intimate with one another (5). The more recent work of Gilligan shows that males and females develop differently in terms of moral expectations and intimacy (6). As a result, people marry with different expectations of their role and behavior as marital partners. Social and cultural factors and demands exert additional influence on these expectations. Theories and ideals that seemed practical and feasible before marriage are often not so afterwards. Reality, of course, is heightened by the pressures of daily concerns about jobs, household chores, bills, and child care. Partnership in marriage, as in business, can be equal or not and agreements may or may not be honored in practice.

Reasons for Marriage

There are many reasons why people marry. The following are the most common, presented in no particular order:

Need for Security

At any age an individual may seek marriage purely in preference to living alone and providing for him- or herself. Such individuals are searching for relief from caring for themselves financially, and sometimes also socially, and require the social security of traditional marriage.

Dependency

Closely linked to a need for security, dependency also includes a giving up of personal responsibility in a psychological sense and relying on another to provide emotional support. Sometimes dependency also includes subservience and the relinquishing of all personal thoughts, ideas, and feelings in favor of those of another who then takes care of all aspects of the relationship. Obviously, there can be varying degrees of dependency from time to time within a marriage, and the need can vary also between different marriages.

Escape

Some marry to escape from difficult home situations when parental quarrels, demands, rules, or financial situations become too overwhelming. This type of marriage is often seen as a socially acceptable and expedient relief and can be used as an escape from other unpleasant circumstances such as unsatisfactory jobs or roommates. Escape as a reason for marriage is often closely linked with dependency and security needs.

Arrangement

Within some families and cultures marriages are still arranged by parents, even within North American society. The young person may have some choice but is still expected to accept the decision of the parents.

Social Pressure

There remains great social pressure on individuals to marry. Single persons find social interactions increasingly difficult as they age. Most activities are organized for couples, especially beyond the teenage years. Persons on their own can become quite lonely, as well as having to deal with well-meaning friends and relatives attempting to match them with someone. Even the couple who have been going out or living together for any length of time are subject to subtle and overt pressures to marry and conform to social expectations.

Pregnancy

A marriage may be precipitated by an unexpected pregnancy. Tolerance for unmarried mothers has not increased in our society enough to allow most young women to bear a child alone. Pregnancy may also be used by one or the other of the couple to force a marriage. The motivations behind this may or may not be conscious at that time.

Desire for a Child

Some marry because they want children and do not find single parenthood acceptable. Here a spouse may be chosen as a good potential parent or gene carrier rather than for any other reason. Once again this motivation for marriage can be linked with any of the others listed here.

Unconscious Need

This is more complicated. Here various factors operate in the choice of a mate, many of which may only reach consciousness much later, or when the marriage is falling apart. These needs can include those left over from childhood or unsatisfactory parenting, self-punishment, rescuing, dependency, mastery, and so on. The chosen spouse has been identified as possessing the necessary characteristics and is a comfortable "fit" (7).

Love

Love has many definitions. In this discussion it is used to describe the reason given merely as a feeling that this is the right person to bring one happiness. Love can operate by itself, as a romantic notion, without regard for any of the other reasons mentioned, or it can combine with any of them.

Completion of One's Self

Following the Eriksonian model of psychosocial development, marriage should be a result of the need for self-completion in a person who has recognized his or her capacity for intimacy and sharing based on a firm personal identity (5). Here marriage would be based on an ability to maintain a commitment to sharing one's self and another's self. Once again, many other factors can operate in conjunction with this.

The Process of Marriage

Whatever the reasons for the marriage, most expect it to last and do not expect to divorce. However, many individuals marry without comprehending what is involved in keeping a marriage together. They often have not thought beyond the fairy-tale ending, "they lived happily ever after." Nor do they ever consider what it takes to do so. Many will not have had a well-functioning parental marriage or any other cohesive family situation to use as a model. They marry with ideas—both conscious and unconscious—of how it should be, but without any notion of how to achieve their dreams.

Having entered marriage, each with their own dreams and expectations, the partners are further shaped by life events and stressors. "Happily ever after" is beset with pressures from work at home and outside, from friends and family, from financial situations, from children, and so on. Maintaining the relationship requires continuous work throughout all these extraneous events and influences, while each partner continues to develop his or her own individual needs and wants. Learning to share and to compromise can be difficult work, and in some situations, the demands can be beyond the person's adaptive capabilities (8).

Here perceptions of roles within marriage and within society become involved. Ideas that were similar in theory before marriage may diverge after the couple have been living together or have become parents. Factors related to the earlier discussion of women's place in today's sociocultural environment are important here.

The wife may assume that she will continue her independent occupational existence and that her partner will continue his, while both share the work of the household. This may be easily feasible until a child enters the relationship. Then social acceptability allows maternity but usually not paternity leave. Likewise, when the child is ill, the mother is allowed to stay at home from her job, but the father is not. Slowly the roles become more traditional. In some marriages, one partner expects the traditional while the other does not; this also may evolve gradually.

The Belittling Process

A couple may begin their life together with mutual expectations of traditional roles. Over the years, the wife often begins to search for new activities as she becomes aware of chronic dissatisfaction with her lifestyle. Initially she may take up hobbies, volunteer work, or adult education courses. More recently, this stage is being bypassed altogether, with the wife commencing to work part- or full-time. Soon these interests are keeping her outside the home for longer and longer periods.

In broadening her sphere the wife quickly moves beyond depending for emotional support and satisfaction only on her husband and children. She feels happier and more content. However, she also feels weary at times, since she still does everything in the home as well. The husband encourages her new interests as long as she maintains her work in the home. However, gradually, as she becomes more self-reliant and assertive, he attempts to revert to the previous situation in the marriage. These attempts are invariably unsuccessful and often lead to the "belittling process."

The belittling process has, of course, as its underlying cause the female–male role dilemma (9). As the wife seeks to assert herself as a "full person" and at the same time to retain, strengthen, and enhance her femininity, the husband attempts to reduce this new assertiveness within parameters of what he desires "his" wife to be. Today, when the wife's new assertiveness often manifests as professional competence, academic ability, or other traits equal to, and often greater than, the husband's, the real role conflict circle is completed. At that stage the marriage partnership is invariably in serious trouble unless the husband is willing to make some very clear and obvious choices.

However, at first, as the belittling proceeds, husbands often win the battle right there. As the wife's efforts and achievements increase, her partner's anxiety is raised commensurately. The wife's success, be it in a profession, studies, or public service, will now be reactively belittled by the husband, who is suddenly uncertain of his role. He is in turmoil, not only because of the changes in his marriage partner, but also the changes expected of him.

These reactions inevitably arouse guilt in the wife while she struggles to maintain the autonomy she has achieved. However, old patterns of trying to please and avoiding anger are difficult to eradicate and quickly surface with the husband's guilt-inducing behavior (10). The wife experiences increasing ambivalence about further autonomous growth. This intermediate stage may pass rather quickly or may last for some years.

The woman's desire for self-fulfillment may continue to gain strength, perhaps encouraged by the support of others or by her own vocational success. As this happens, anger at her husband's behavior intensifies within. It is at this time that some women seek the help of a psychotherapist, frequently with an initial complaint of anxiety or depression (see case examples at end of this chapter). In any case, the husband at this point often cannot tolerate the process any further and may face several difficult problems. He may become depressed. He may decide to leave the marriage and turn to another woman, often younger than his wife. This woman may have already established her personal and occupational identity and he may find that he can tolerate in her what he could not in his wife. Or he may turn to a woman more content with the traditional life, a woman much like his wife when he first married her!

As Miller wrote (11), a loving relationship can be very satisfying and can increase one's self-worth if one partner is not seen as inferior to the other. When the woman's position is belittled and her feelings disregarded, a relationship becomes unpleasantly complicated and begins to unravel with difficult consequences for all involved. Thus, the belittling process is clearly a product of our sociocultural expectations of men and women and their continuing evolution throughout this century.

It goes almost without saying that modern socioeconomic pressures exacerbate the problem. Many women who have entered the workforce do so out of necessity in order to provide more for their families. Success and achievement, after entry into the workforce, are often a byproduct. In general, it appears that when women in the workforce confine themselves to less important positions, where they are simply regarded as an additional wage earner, there is less chance of the belittling process. However, as soon as the woman starts to reach her true potential of achievement, her marriage partner often feels threatened. This is worsened by the situation, so prevalent today, in which the husband may be unemployed and the wife becomes the sole breadwinner. This type of "role reversal" is very far from general acceptance.

Yet society has changed considerably, particularly since the end of World War II. The modern "dual career" family is today the norm rather than the exception, although even here the dual roles are far from equal. Even highly motivated dual career marriage partners can experience the belittling process when demands for greater equality in the marriage are combined with inordinate success in the wife's career.

It has been argued that the real answers must be found in the wider establishment of the true "equalitarian family" (12). This has been defined as a family in which the marriage partners have equal rights and duties prescribed both at the societal and dyadic levels (12). It should, however, be noted that terms such as *equality* and *equity* in their true constructive meaning, without their emotive basis, appear to be much more widely accepted at the societal than at the social level. For example, the legal rights and duties of the marriage partners relating to functions such as procreation, socialization of offspring, economic questions, and physical welfare are relatively clear today. The aberrations still in existence are quickly being eroded (although fundamentalist religions have defended the status quo). However, these changes are only in response to the slow evolutionary changes in gender roles that have filtered through from the societal to the political decision-making level.

On the other hand, we must treat these welcome changes with extreme caution. As we know so well from the phenomenon of racial discrimination, to change the law to enforce greater equality is one thing, but to force society to change its attitudes, which are the cause of the inequality in the first place, is quite another. In the belittling process, the wife may well be "equal" to her husband before the law but not in his perception.

Women are now fulfilling roles previously closed to them. While society and its laws have changed over the decades, the traditional norms of marriage have had difficulties accommodating these shifts. A traditional marriage is based on inequality, and this becomes manifest when the wife wants to assert her independence or to reach for increased intellectual and personal fulfillment. This leads to marriage breakdown and frequent psychosocial problems that carry through into the divorce process. Thus, during the separation and divorce the belittling that began in the marriage continues and influences and interferes in the decision making just as it overwhelmed the marriage itself.

Divorce

The pressures described above can lead to marriage breakdown and divorce (13). Often a woman who would not have contemplated this drastic step while still dependent will not feel free to break this "chain." She will realize that the belittling process, which degrades her feelings, will cease only if she returns to a more traditional role in the family or leaves the family altogether. Although no hard data on the belittling process as a cause for divorce are available, it can nevertheless be stated quite clearly that a very large percentage of divorces involving "dual career" marriages must fit in this category. For example, a recent major study on the new Canadian divorce legislation commenced its examination of reasons for divorce by stating unequivocally that the combination of fewer children and increased educational opportunities for wives leads to the kind of pressures that cause divorce (14). In particular, as wives are "expected to combine the super-woman careers of having a home and a job, the backup resources of the extended family are no longer available" (14).

In Canada, nearly 40 percent of all marriages end in divorce, and the length of marriages ending in divorce has dropped from 16 years in 1969 to 12 years in 1984 (14). In the United States, these figures are generally higher (15). In examining such statistics, it is relatively easy to conclude that less traditional "dependence" by wives, based on greater personal opportunities, will inevitably lead to marriage breakdown without the tolerance needed in a reasonably equal dual career setting. Very often the belittling process, as a reflection of the husband's uncertainties about the changes in his "successful" wife, is a clear sign of the lack of such tolerance or the inability to accept change.

However, at this stage the belittling process can be even more invidious. Often the wife has been a "model" traditional wife, mother, and homemaker for a number of years. She finds, usually in early middle age, with the children nearly grown or departed, that she can no longer be simply a "homemaker." She may go back to work full- or part-time, she may undertake academic or vocational studies, or she may go into business. Often this is tolerated, perhaps initially even encouraged, by the husband, until the threat of the wife's success in her new endeavors becomes apparent. This is when the first stage of the belittling process is most apparent. Unless the wife is willing to retreat from her new goals, and many do, marriage breakdown is almost inevitable. Yet in societal terms these pressures have only been barely recognized in the development of new divorce legislation.

In Western legal terms, despite a number of reforms, marriage and divorce legislation still provides a basis for the so-called traditional values. As a result, a number of advocates for more equitable feminine roles argue that there is an indirect, yet clear relationship between law and the oppression of women (16). Furthermore, it is also argued that this link is aided and abetted by marital and divorce legislation as it exists today. Although there have been some perceptible changes, there is also considerable evidence that these arguments have merit.

The Canadian divorce law of 1986 is one of the most up-to-date laws in the world. It attempts to simplify and modernize a system that was considered out of date even prior to World War II. The grounds for divorce are reduced from 15 to the single ground that a divorce will be granted upon an application of either one or both marriage partners that there has been a breakdown in the marriage (17, 18). Such breakdown can be proved only by establishing that

1. The spouses have lived separate and apart for at least one year immediately prior to the commencement of the proceedings; or
2. The spouse against whom the proceedings are brought has, since the celebration of the marriage, committed adultery, or treated the other spouse with physical or mental cruelty of such a kind as to render intolerable the continued cohabitation of the spouses (18).

Unfortunately, the retention of the need for proof of marital breakdown has also preserved the adversarial nature of the proceedings. However, it is conceded that today the adversial nature of divorce proceedings is often superseded by the bitter battles relating to custody and property divisions. It is also here that the belittled wife faces some of her most difficult problems.

If the wife finds that she can meet the mental cruelty criterion, which under the law must be "weighty and grave"—that is, more than the ordinary wear and tear of family life, amounting to more than temporary incompatibility—she can make her case for a divorce (19, 20). However, the test for such cruelty is subjective, and she would have to chronicle how the belittling process made further cohabitation intolerable. This is an area wide open for court bias. It is not inconceivable that a male judge, faced by a husband arguing that the wife abandoned traditional familial roles, will be less sympathetic to the wife. At this stage even the woman's hard-won success may backfire. She may have to contribute some of her holdings, particularly in jurisdictions where marital property is split, upon marriage dissolution. Or she may lose custody over children upon argument that she is too busy in her career, studies, or business. She may be given custody over children plus a settlement which may well be insufficient to cover the costs involved. This may then involve her in lengthy and frustrating maintenance battles which are prevalent in all jurisdictions these days. Even more inequitably, she may be deprived of her rightful share of her husband's holdings on the grounds that as a successful woman she can now take care of herself! As a result, she may find herself, in middle age, divorced, quite alone, with limited means and only on the threshold of a new life. The adversarial nature of the divorce, custody, and property settlement process will thus ensure that the husband's bitterness, which was the root cause of the belittling process, is perpetuated through the divorce proceedings.

Although a number of feminists argue eloquently that these problems can be removed through radical family law reform, it is doubtful if any law can be so designed at this stage (19, 20). The law is often accused of being unresponsive to perceived societal requirements, of being ultraconservative in approach, of changing too slowly, of being too inflexible to the point of harshness, of catering only to the lowest common denominator of social demand, and so on. All of this is probably true to a great extent, yet such accusations ignore the fact that the law is not a self-developing, monolithic structure, although it can easily be perceived as such, but simply a system that responds to sociopolitical demands. Therefore, it is society and the political system that must bring about changes in the law. In the area of family law, rightly or wrongly, such changes have not been deemed to be required. Any changes that do occur are thus far from the radical innovations often demanded.

On the other hand, in many jurisdictions divorce laws have at least attempted to create greater equity between the spouses on marriage breakup. Property division, more adequate maintenance orders, and periodic revision of changed financial circumstances have placed women in particular in a better position. Nevertheless, as already indicated, the continued adversarial nature of all these proceedings ensures that the belittling process continues. First, the embittered husband, even—at times especially—if well positioned financially, will fight lengthy legal battles in order to prevent a more equitable settlement. It matters not if this battle is often waged at great cost, benefitting only the legal professionals involved. While the fight rages, the wife is often left in difficult circumstances, having to contest an expensive legal dispute with few ready means and a home and children to maintain. Even if she wins, it is often a Pyrrhic victory, because the enforcement of maintenance orders is very problematic. For example, a recent report states that in one jurisdiction some 85 percent of all maintenance orders are not followed (21). This figure is not very different in many other jurisdictions. In many instances this is a continuation of the belittling process—perhaps further escalated by the inevitable bitterness of the divorce proceeding itself. It is not at all unusual for the ex-husband to prefer personal financial ruin to proper maintenance of his children and former wife. If the former wife has moved into a successful career or business of her own, she will usually have great difficulties obtaining any maintenance for the children and will obtain none for herself, even in cases where the husband still holds property that was mutually built up during the marriage.

Eventually though, the woman will extricate herself from her former life and assume her new role and identity. Often the scars of the lengthy belittling period are very deep and the help of the psychotherapist may be particularly important even at this stage. The woman has come through 10 stages of the belittling process. These stages can take months, but often take years. They are

1. Initial objection of the husband to the wife's independence and ambitions;
2. Escalation of the initial objection;
3. Serious disputes in the marriage—this is the "your job or me" stage;
4. Estrangement;
5. Separation, often with legal implications;
6. Commencement of divorce proceedings;
7. Divorce proceedings, including custody and maintenance applications;
8. Final decree stage of the divorce;
9. Enforcement of divorce orders;
10. Postdivorce stage.

Although the problems faced by the woman in the belittling journey are clearly exacerbated during the legal stages, the overall process is not within the jurisprudential dimension. It is a complex reflection of unresolved interpersonal problems between marriage partners in a societal setting that has not yet come to terms with women's greater search for individual identity and full potential. Until such search is given its rightful place in society the therapist and the lawyer are simply peripheral participants in an unequal process.

Case Examples

Case Example 1

Mrs. A, 46 years old, complained of depressive symptoms that were immobilizing. She had depended on the strong support of her mother and sister-in-law to manage her daily existence ever since her husband had suddenly, and without notice, left her and filed for divorce. She had three children: a daughter, 24, who was working in another city, and sons, age 22 and 20, at home. Mrs. A had married at age 19 her 20-year-old long-time boyfriend. She worked as a secretary while he completed his professional training. Once the first child was born Mrs. A remained at home. Through the years she devoted herself to the home, children, and her husband's career. He became successful in his work and politically and socially influential. They were very active socially together. She gave up her own personal interests early in the marriage to share his.

Known in the community as a pleasant and gregarious man, at home he was often ill-tempered and occasionally hit her. She was blamed for any difficulty he encountered and was constantly told how stupid she was. He managed all of their financial matters and made all major decisions. One evening he returned home from work, berated her when he could not find something of his, announced to her he was leaving and did so immediately.

During the divorce negotiations and proceedings, he continued to treat her with contempt and harassments. She gradually discovered, by hiring detectives, that he was living with his secretary. This woman was slightly younger, very assertive, and independent. Following the divorce he suddenly also left that relationship and shortly thereafter married another woman. The new wife had her own occupation, which she left upon marrying him. He in turn gave up his social and political activities to spend time with her. However, he continued to regularly institute new legal challenges against Mrs. A, especially as she became self-sufficient and independent.

Case Example 2

Mrs. B, 38 years old, complained of inordinate rage at her 40-year-old estranged husband, who was living with another woman aged 22. She felt his behavior toward her and their three children was inconsiderate and financially unfair as they proceeded toward a divorce. Mrs. B saw herself as having to battle for a fair share of their assets at a time when she should have been comfortable and secure.

This couple had been together through college, where Mr. B had been a well-known sports hero and she an admired student leader and fraternity queen. After graduating she had worked as a teacher to support them as he went through a professional school. Near graduation she had become pregnant, and the next two children had been born during Mr. B's further postgraduate training. They had lived frugally on borrowed money for those several years, she spending most nights and weekends alone with the children and he studying and training.

They had looked forward to returning to their home town and to having time together then.

However, once home Mr. B had remained very busy establishing his new career. At first Mrs. B had been occupied with their new home and settling the children into schools. Then she had begun to do volunteer work with some charitable groups and social organizations. Growing more confident of her abilities, Mrs. B. had returned to university and completed graduate school, while continuing to run their home and care for their growing children. Mr. B had remained occupied with his work and many sports activities. He had complained when his wife was unavailable when he wanted her to prepare meals and subtly discouraged her studies. They were doing little together. His disparagement had increased when she found a part-time employment in her new field.

Matters had improved for a year or so when she had interested him in beginning a small business with another couple. They had been together more often, but then he had begun to spend time at his sports again and to be disinterested in her. She had begun an affair with another man, deliberately hoping to reinterest her husband. Instead he had become enraged and left. The children had been 17, 16, and 13 at the time. Soon thereafter he had met and begun to live with a 22-year-old woman who had quickly become pregnant. The young woman had a busy full-time career which she maintained while sharing his sports activities. In turn he spent more time at home with her. Mr. B and Mrs. B fought bitterly over the division of their considerable assets, and he portrayed himself as poor and financially insolvent as a result.

Case Example 3

Mrs. C, 27 years old, complained that her husband was depressed and she was looking for help for him. They had been married four years and had a one-year-old child. He worked as a foreman and union representative; she was an office clerk-secretary. Mr. C was an only child whose mother had devoted herself to her housework and cooking for her husband and son. Mrs. C was the youngest and the only girl in a family in which both parents worked outside the home and she had been expected to help out from an early age, although her brother had not.

Mrs. and Mrs. C had lived together for a year before marrying, and all had gone smoothly until the baby was born. Mrs. C found it increasingly difficult to manage her job, care for the baby, and keep the house tidy. Mr. C did not share the household tasks because he held a second job most nights. He felt that his wife should be able to organize her time in order to do all her jobs. He thought and said that she was untidy, lazy, disorganized, and stupid. Mrs. C was unaccustomed to arguing and used to acquiescing to and pleasing others. She began to overeat and gain weight and spent money carelessly. He grew more and more worried about debt because he wanted to save for a house of their own. He questioned every dollar she spent but demanded she pay all of their bills.

Mrs. C slowly resumed some old hobbies, but Mr. C resented the time she spent on them instead of doing housework. He became depressed and very irritable. She became tearful and more passively resistant. They began to discuss separation.

These cases illustrate the belittling process as outlined in this chapter. It differs from that which can occur within any form of relationship, such as the constant demeaning of one person by another. Instead it is a husband's belittling of his wife's vocational and personal achievements as she moves from a more traditional role into one of greater equality. This difficulty in accepting her will often pervade the divorce process as well.

References

1. Woloch N: Women and the American Experience. New York, Alfred A. Knopf, 1984
2. Solomon BM: In the Company of Educated Women. New Haven, CT, Yale University Press, 1985
3. Friedan B: The Feminine Mystique, New York, Norton, 1963
4. Friedan B: The Second Stage. New York, Summit, 1981
5. Erikson E: Identity, Youth and Crisis. New York, Norton, 1968

6. Gilligan C: In a Different Voice. Cambridge, MA, Harvard University Press, 1982
7. Money J: Love Maps. New York, Irvington, 1986
8. Jacobson GF: Power dynamics in love and marriage, Psychiatric Annals 16:647-649, 1986
9. Gold JH, Gold E: The belittled wife: social, legal and psychotherapeutic considerations. Can J Psychiatry 26:402-405, 1981
10. Horney K: The problem of feminine masochism. Psychoanal Rev 22:241-257, 1935
11. Miller JB: Sexual inequality: men's dilemma. Am J Psychoanal 32:147-155, 1972
12. Eichler M: The equalitarian family in Canada, in Marriage, Family and Society. Edited by SP Wakil. Toronto, Butterworth, 1975
13. Rabkin B: Loving and Leaving. Toronto, McClelland and Stewart, 1985
14. Bissett-Johnson A, Day DC: The New Divorce Law—A Commentary on the Divorce Act 1985. Toronto, Carswell, 1985
15. Kessler S: The American Way of Divorce. Chicago, Nelson-Hall, 1975
16. Smart C: The Ties That Bind—Law, Marriage and the Reproduction of Patriarchal Relations. London, Routledge & Kegan Paul, 1984
17. The 1968 Canadian Divorce Act. S.C. 1967-68, c.24; R.S.C. 1970, c.D-8
18. Divorce Act, 1985, S.C. 1986, c.4, s.8(2)
19. Davies C: Family Law in Canada. Toronto, Carswell, 1984
20. LeBrocq v. LeBrocq (1964) 3 A11E.R.464 (C.A.)
21. 85% default on support payments. Ottawa Citizen, January 24, 1987

Chapter 3

Assessing and Treating Divorcing Men

MICHAEL F. MYERS, M.D., F.R.C.P.(C)

Assessing and Treating Divorcing Men

Although the divorce rate in the United States had been beginning to fall, in 1985 it crept up again by 2 percent to a rate of 5 divorces per 1,000 people (1). Hence, marital separation continues to be a major stressor that affects all family members. There is now considerable psychiatric literature on the impact of divorce on children (2–6), on women (7–9), and increasingly on men (10–14). This chapter focuses on issues that are important to keep in mind when assessing and treating divorcing men who present for psychiatric assistance.

First, sociological research has demonstrated that there are sex differences in divorce: Men have higher psychiatric morbidity rates and mortality rates (15, 16). Bloom (17) noted high first-time psychiatric hospital admission rates for separated men, especially newly separated men. Jacobs's (12) study of divorcing fathers revealed that the threatened loss of their relationships with their children is frequently the presenting complaint of men in the midst of a divorce crisis. More recently, Jacobs (18) wrote about the "involuntary child absence" syndrome in fathers, which he described as the group of symptoms, feelings, ideas, and behaviors that are precipitated in some parents during or following separation or divorce when they are threatened with, feel threatened by, or must in fact live with a minimal or diminished relationship or no relationship at all with one or more of their children.

Divorcing and divorced fathers have been studied more extensively than divorced men who are childless (10, 12, 19, 20). Such research has focused specifically on the father's postdivorce adjustment, the farther-child relationship in pre- and postdivorce situations, noncustodial fathers, and single fathers. Most data suggest that those fathers who have continued contact and involvement with their children after separation are less depressed. Furthermore, one cannot always predict the nature and quality of the postseparation fathering by the relationship during the marriage: Some "closely involved" fathers before separation do not maintain this behavior after separation because of their inability to adapt to visitation status (10, 20). Other men become active and interested fathers only after separation.

Case Example 1

Mr. and Mrs. A. had been married for 15 years and had two sons aged 12 and 7 when they came for marital therapy. Both were extremely unhappy with each other and had been for several years. They had a number of concerns that they bickered about: Mr. A.'s alcoholism and his refusal to do anything about it; Mrs. A.'s morbid obesity and their 7-year-old's increasing weight gain; lack of sexual interest in each other; economic reversals the previous two years; and Mr. A.'s intrusive parents. Although they were very unhappy as a couple and rarely did anything together, each of them was superb at parenting and respected the other's involvement with the children.

During marital therapy, Mrs. A. decided she wanted to separate from Mr. A. unless he agreed to go to Alcoholics Anonymous (Mrs. A. had been attending Alanon for the previous year). As in the past, Mr. A. refused, and after a couple of weeks he agreed to move out of the family home. He took a small basement apartment not far away so he could be close to his children.

Like many newly separated couples, their visitation arrangement with the children began on quite a friendly and unstructured basis. Mr. A. spent parts of several evenings and weekends at the family home and occasionally had one or both children overnight at his apartment. However, as weeks passed, Mrs. A. began feeling increasingly territorial about the family home—and she was now dating. Negotiations were attempted to establish a more structured and predictable visitation schedule centered at Mr. A.'s residence. Although his finances were now better, he refused to take a larger apartment where he could more easily have the children for visits overnight, once during the week and one weekend night. He was adjusting to a new job and also dating; he argued that he didn't want to be "pinned down" to specific visitation days.

Several months passed. Mrs. A. became concerned about her oldest son's mood and behavior. She felt he was both depressed and angry about the separation. Mr. A.'s requests to see the children were fewer and unpredictable, and on two occasions he cancelled at the last minute. The boys often left messages on his answering machine that were not returned. He withdrew from therapy as well, promising to still see the children but stating he was very busy. His contacts with his sons remained infrequent.

Case Example 2

Dr. and Mrs. B. requested separation therapy. They had decided to separate only recently and had not yet told their children, ages 7 and 5. They had questions regarding how to tell the children, what to tell them, and when to tell them. Dr. B. wanted a joint custody arrangement on an alternating week-long basis. Mrs. B. was aghast. She not only saw herself as the primary parent but also described Dr. B. as "in another world this past year." By this she meant that he was rarely home before the kids were in bed and he played sports all weekend with his male friends. Dr. B. did not disagree; he argued that he was out a lot deliberately because of the tension and unhappiness at home.

Mrs. B. was willing to give the arrangement a trial period of six weeks. Although she was not optimistic, she admitted that she welcomed being freed up a bit from bearing almost total responsibility for the children. She felt guilty about letting down her partners in her law firm the previous year; she also felt the children needed their father more. Six weeks later things were going well. Mrs. B.'s only complaint was how much she missed daily contact with the children when they were at Dr. B.'s home (a complaint which is universal in joint custody arrangements). Dr. B. was very happy with shared parenting and admitted "I feel I've returned to the land of the living." Their arrangement continued to work well and was formalized eventually in their divorce decree.

Routes to Treatment

Most marital breakdowns are characterized by extremely complex, multidetermined, and ambiguous issues. Attempting to analyze "who left whom" as a significant variable is difficult. In fact, in many cases, this may be actually confusing, misleading, or reductionistic. Nevertheless, for a subgroup of divorcing couples, one party assumes the initiator role in the separation process, and this has implications for help seeking.

Thus we can examine three separation situations—husband initiated, wife initiated, and mutually initiated—and the routes to treatment.

Husband Initiated

In husband-initiated separations, the husband has come to the decision to leave his wife. This decision may vary in its duration and conviction. He may request treatment and come with her. His main emotion may be anxiety about his wife's mental health after the separation, and part of his motivation for treatment may be to align his wife with the therapist in order to alleviate his guilt. Many of these men will have already mourned their marriages and are well into being emotionally separate. Some will be involved with a new partner. In general, such men are not severely symptomatic.

Case Example 3

When Mr. and Mrs. C. came for marital therapy, Mrs. C. was three months pregnant with their third child. Mr. C. was very definite and forthright in his manner. He stated that he was planning to separate very soon, that he was miserable in his marriage, and that if he didn't leave soon, he'd "go bananas." Although Mrs. C.'s pregnancy made him feel even more guilty about separating, he resented her for not agreeing to have a therapeutic abortion. Mrs. C. was heartbroken and devastated.

She loved her husband intensely, was completely against separating, and was also completely against abortion.

Mr. C. left that evening. Both were in individual therapy for several months. Mr. C. began to feel much better immediately. He was relieved to have both a therapist and an obstetrician looking after his wife. His active involvement with his children was especially important as Mrs. C. became quite depressed for the first two months of the separation and functioned poorly. Once the baby was born she was increasingly able to come to terms with being on her own and to accept the loss of her husband.

Wife Initiated

In wife-initiated separation, the wife has decided to leave her husband. She may present for treatment on her own, fearful of what the separation might do to her husband. Or, as in the previous case, she may come in with her husband so that she can arrange a therapist for him before leaving. Despite her husband's interest in marital therapy, she wants assistance only with separating. Those men who come for help on their own, either while their wives are preparing to leave or after their wives have already left, are generally struggling with abandonment. Elsewhere (14, 21) I have described in some detail the symptomatic profile and underlying dynamics of such men and aspects of treatment with them. They may be very symptomatic, in some cases extremely suicidal or homicidal, and require very careful assessment and management.

Case Example 4

Mr. D., a 36-year-old teacher, came for therapy because of despondency, a 15-pound weight loss, severe sleep disturbance, inability to concentrate on his work, frequent headaches, and uncontrollable crying spells. He had daily thoughts of suicide and death wishes. "The only reason I haven't killed myself is because of my children," he stated. He had been living alone since he and his wife separated one month earlier. He hoped that the separation would be temporary only. He was given an antidepressant and told to return in one week.

Mrs. D. called the following day and requested to be seen alone regarding her marriage and separation. With Mr. D.'s consent, a visit was arranged with her. She was relieved that he had come to see a psychiatrist because she was very worried about him. When she had told him initially six months earlier that she wanted to separate, he had threatened suicide a number of times. She had decided not to leave then but continued in her resolve to separate eventually, as had happened. Since living apart he had made veiled references to harming her and the children and then to committing suicide. She wanted the therapist to know that her father-in-law had committed suicide. She was certain that the marriage was over, that it had been for years, but that she did not feel confident enough until recently to try making it on her own.

Mutually Initiated

In mutually initiated separations, both the husband and wife consciously desire to separate. They usually request and present for treatment together. Predominant emotions are sadness and varying amounts of anxiety about being alone. It is important to note that the mutuality may be only a surface contract. One of the partners may be much clearer and more desirous of separation than the other, who may be highly ambivalent and perhaps covertly quite symptomatic. A therapist must be watchful of underdiagnosing some of these couples.

Case Example 5

Mr. and Mrs. E., married for 12 years and childless by choice, came for marital therapy "to see if we should remain together or not." They presented a calm, united front of having a friendly relationship, "like brother and sister," but lacking in both sexual and nonsexual affection. They had ceased sexual relations together about five years previously. In the interim both had had "brief liaisons," outside the marriage, for which neither admitted to feelings of jealousy, hurt, or threat.

After the first visit Mrs. E. announced that she was moving out. "It's time to take the plunge," she said. Mr. E. agreed. Neither felt the need to continue therapy. Four months later, Mr. E.

called, worried about his wife, saying that she was getting mixed up with the wrong crowd, setting herself up to get hurt, and so forth. He came in and was found to be quite depressed. He admitted that he was eating poorly, drinking more than usual, and was isolated socially. After a few supportive visits, he began to feel better about being on his own. He was dating someone and felt happy about that. He stopped worrying about Mrs. E.

About six months later, Mrs. E. called with a similar story, that she was worried about Mr. E. and "his new life style." When seen, she was openly mourning her marriage and what once was. She had had several short-term relationships, none of them satisfactory. She had asked her husband if there might be a chance for a reconciliation at some point, but he told her he thought not.

Clinical Findings

Divorce hurts, and the degree of this hurt varies from one person to the next. The intensity, the duration, and the modulation also depend on many other factors: the individual's ego strength; vulnerability and predisposition to loss; cultural and ethnic group; religious affiliation or lack thereof; socioeconomic level; age and stage of life; and, as stated before, the sex of the individual. Divorce is a process, not an event. Psychiatrists see divorcing people at various stages of mourning; most will be struggling with aspects of denial, anger and protest, bargaining, and depression (22). Some or all of the following symptoms can be expected: anxiety, sleep disturbance, somatization, bewilderment and disorganization, grief, and clinical depression. Diagnoses may include a wide range of syndromes: phase of life problem, various adjustment disorders, somatoform disorders, anxiety states, phobic disorders, affective disorders, and substance use disorders (23).

What has been described here are symptoms that can occur in any divorcing individual regardless of sex. What about men? Are there findings that are specific to men? In my practice, men at various stages of marital separation and divorce have displayed the following: drug and alcohol abuse and dependency; violent behavior toward others, especially their wives; diminished work efficiency, including absences from work; compulsive and frenetic dating; indiscriminate sexual behavior with women, including first-time involvement with prostitutes; and early entry into new relationships. This last observation is in keeping with the research finding that men remarry earlier than women and also remarry at a greater rate (24).

Case Example 6

Dr. F., a 32-year-old emergency room physician, came for therapy with a chief complaint of "I'm worried about my morals." This man and his wife had separated six months earlier after seven years of marriage and two young children, ages 4 and 2. Dr. F. visited his sons every two or three days at their home and had them every other weekend at his apartment, depending on his work schedule. This was going well. "It's when I'm not with the boys that I'm at loose ends," he stated.

Dr. F. went on to describe how restless, agitated, and panicky he became after work or at other times when he did not have something scheduled. He said that although he had the reputation of being "this year's most eligible bachelor" at his tennis club, and although he had dated many women since separating, he did not feel good about himself. He always felt preoccupied, hated being at home alone, and on a number of occasions awoke in the night feeling "in a panic." He would get up, pace, get dressed, and go out for a drive. On several occasions, he had picked up a prostitute, had sex in his car, and ended up feeling horrible about himself afterwards. Despite his fear of disease, especially AIDS, the behavior continued unchecked.

Dr. F. did very well with supportive and exploratory psychotherapy. There were clearly decipherable psychodynamic determinants of his symptomatology. Once these were uncovered and worked through, he felt better. He had suffered from separation anxiety when faced with loss since his parents' divorce when he was seven years old. Being able to ventilate openly and frankly in a therapeutic relationship was especially helpful for him.

Another common finding in men who are divorcing is isolation. This has implications for treatment and colors the transference. Many separated men are emotionally remote from their families of origin, and few have close male friends with whom they are verbally and emotionally intimate about their situation. Those men who do reach out to their male friends may report that they are not that helpful and may feel rebuffed by them. In many respects, this is not surprising: North American men in general do not tend to have close and long-standing friendships with men outside their marriages. Levinson, in an in-depth study of men throughout the life cycle, noted that "In our interviews, friendship was largely noticeable by its absence" (25). Some divorcing men have platonic friendships with women that provide sustenance and companionship.

Case Example 7

Mr. and Mrs. G. began conjoint marital work, although Mrs. G. was beyond working on her marriage. After three visits her husband was more able to recognize and accept her position as the two of them discussed separation. This continued for a couple more visits, at the end of which Mr. G. expressed his desire to continue in therapy alone after separation. Mrs. G. felt fine handling things on her own.

Mr. G. was seen about every two weeks for three months after the separation. He responded well to support. Part of the therapeutic focus was to encourage him to open up more with his brothers, who lived in the same community, and with his male friends. This was difficult for him and he did not receive a lot of encouragement from them either. One brother accused him of "being gripped in self-pity," and the other did not show up for the lunch that they had planned together. He played squash regularly with his two closest friends, but he actively resisted talking much about being separated. Nor did his friends ask how he was doing.

At the end of one session during which he had awkwardly and embarrassingly described some sexual timidity with a woman he was seeing, he warmly shook my hand and said, "I can't tell you how much it helps to come here.... You've become my best friend." Many male patients have said this, and it points, sadly, to the problems that many men have being intimate with other men.

It is wise to remember that many separated men will not be sharing their private, inner feelings with anyone. Some are terrified or are repelled by the thought of returning to an empty apartment alone after work; they go to bars and eat dinner in restaurants. Some are still in love with their wives and fantasize about being back together. Despite bravado, many feel awkward in meeting and dating new women. Relationships are characterized by approach/avoidance behaviors and fears of intimacy. There may be a plethora of sexual worries: frank avoidance, mechanical sex devoid of feeling, guilt associated with sex, performance anxiety, various sexual dysfunctions, a subjective sense of being "over the hill," and feelings of intimidation by younger men.

Case Example 8

Mr. H., a 41-year-old contractor, was seen 18 months after he and his wife separated. His chief complaint was in not being able to sustain an erection. Mr. H. began having erectile difficulties the first time he attempted sex with another woman (he had never had sexual difficulties with his wife) about nine months after separation. He rationalized that he did not know the woman very well and had had too much alcohol. However, the same difficulty had occurred since with three other women when he had not been drinking, and he was now sufficiently worried and lacking in confidence that he sought professional help.

Mr. H.'s personal and family history was significant. He was a very conservative and conscientious man whose father was a minister and mother a teacher. He and his wife met in high school, dated for several years, and married when they were both 23. They "petted" before marriage but nothing more. Neither had ever dated anyone else. Their sexual relationship was fine after working at it together the first year or two of marriage. He had never been sexually active outside his marriage with anyone else.

The demise of Mr. H.'s marriage was extremely upsetting, came without warning to him, and was important psychodynamically in contributing to his sexual dysfunction. During the last year of his marriage he had sensed that his wife "seemed different." He had felt that she was becoming increasingly remote and private. When confronted about this, she had denied anything was amiss. As she socialized more and more without him and was increasingly oblique regarding her whereabouts, he had suspected she was involved with someone else, which she denied. One night he deliberately returned a day earlier from a business trip and found her with another man in their home. After several weeks of discussion, including a few visits with a marital therapist, the two of them had separated, against Mr. H.'s wishes. He still loved his wife but she was very ambivalent and also felt she needed to pursue her new relationship. This she did and began living with this man about six months later.

Mr. H. had enormous unfinished business regarding his marriage and separation. He had not adequately mourned and was not in touch with much anger or resentment about the end of his marriage. He blamed himself almost entirely for his wife's meeting someone else. He was extremely vulnerable to repeated hurt, did not trust easily, and had very little confidence about himself as a man, let alone as a lover. In fact, he was not conscious of the fact that his overall sexual drive was suppressed, not just his erectile ability. He began to feel better after 10 to 12 psychotherapy visits. His capacity for intimacy, sexual expression, and commitment to a new relationship gradually improved and he became comfortable in a relationship with a woman he had met through mutual friends.

Treatment

Psychotherapy Training Issues

Trainees tend to underdiagnose the psychiatric distress of some men, especially younger men, in the midst of a divorce crisis. In some cases, this is clearly attributable to the student's lack of clinical experience. In other cases, it is due to denial and an inability to comprehend the magnitude of pain that can occur in a young man due to loss of a love object. One male junior resident stated, "I can't understand why he's so depressed. He's mired in self-pity. Hell, he's young, he's good-looking, he's got a good job—there're all kinds of women out there if he'd only get off his butt and meet some of them!"

On the other hand, those trainees who themselves have been married and divorced (or who have had committed relationships end) seem to have a greater empathic understanding. One medical student, while discussing his patient, suddenly became tearful, then embarrassed and apologetic. He explained, "I asked the patient about suicidal thoughts. He said no but that everyday he just wants to die. Boy, could I identify with him! For weeks after my girlfriend and I broke up, I just wanted to die. And how lonely I felt with those feelings—I thought I was going crazy. I didn't tell anyone. I cover up well. Just like this guy. Whew!"

Nowadays many medical students and residents are themselves adult "children of divorce." They have experienced first hand much of what their patients are describing and may therefore have a heightened sensitivity to marital and separation dynamics. However, some may have unresolved issues around their parents' divorce that if unrecognized will get in the way.

Case Example 9

Sam, a 24-year-old senior medical student, complained of feelings of anxiety and depression after completing his clerkship in psychiatry. He had not only clashed with his clinical supervisor but also received an evaluation that was below average in grade. He was furious and terribly disappointed because he was considering psychiatry as a career. His supervisor described him as "an angry young man whose affect alienates those around him"; "he lacks clinical neutrality in his work—on one occasion he insulted the husband of one of his patients"; "he likes psychiatry but he's inconsistent—he reads too much psychopathology into Patient A and normalizes everything about Patient B."

Sam had a lot of insight into his difficulties and knew that he needed psychotherapy. His parents separated when he was 13, one week after his Bar Mitzvah. Twelve years later he still could not talk about it without crying, and he never felt that he really understood what had happened, despite repeated attempts on his part to get an explanation from each of his parents. His previously close relationship with his father was lost and never recaptured since his father later remarried and started a second family. He was full of unresolved anger toward his father, and he felt a lot of guilt about that. His statement "I just never trusted him again as someone I could count on—in fact, I don't trust any man, any father figure, authority figure, teacher, mentor, no one as someone who is really there for me" summed up his feelings.

After his parents divorced he became "the man of the house" and became closer to and very protective of his mother, who never remarried. It was only during medical school that he began to resent his mother's dependence and not inconsiderable demands on him. He began to feel she undermined his relationships with women and in fact blamed her for his most recent relationship with a classmate not succeeding. This breakup of a two-year cohabiting relationship had occurred just before he began rotation in psychiatry.

Sam was able to connect all of this as contributing to his difficulty with his clinical supervisor, a man, and to his work with his patients. He entered long-term psychotherapy and made tremendous strides in his interpersonal relationships both at work and in his personal life. His self-image and self-worth improved as he became more convinced of his lovableness and worthiness as an adult man. He gained a healthier degree of individuation from his mother and came to accept the limitations in his relationship with his father. He decided against psychiatry and chose family practice, which he enjoys and finds fulfilling.

Issues in Treatment

Men in the midst of a divorce crisis, especially those who feel abandoned, must be very carefully assessed for their suicidal and/or homicidal potential. One must try to gauge the degree of despair and frustration and loneliness. How well or poorly are they doing living on their own? For those men who are back living with parents, how is that for them? If they are drinking, how much and how frequently? Has access to their children been curtailed in any way? Has it been severed? How sorrowful are they? How angry and threatening? Do they own a firearm?

Separation and divorce counseling can be extremely therapeutic for both parties. Seeing both partners together and separately helps the therapist to remain objective and neutral. Knowing and observing each person as the separation evolves enables the therapist to more easily recognize and pinpoint when the partners' expectations of each other are unrealistic. Strong affects can be identified and discharged in a therapeutic setting, which may help to dilute the aggression and potential for violence. Therapeutic concern and hopefulness may counteract feelings of isolation and despair.

In cases in which mothers have sole custody, therapists should examine the relationship that the divorced father has with his child or children closely. Jacobs (11) has urged professionals who do crisis work to be aware of the social, political, and legal issues facing divorcing fathers. In his extensive review of the literature in this field, he highlights findings that a) children deprived of their fathers may suffer from a range of emotional problems and b) divorced fathers often suffer when separated from their children and tend to do better with greater continuity of parent–child contact. Therapists are in a unique position to ensure some balance for all parties involved and to intervene as mediators when necessary.

However, caution is urged in situations in which it appears that the patient, a divorced father, is being treated unfairly by his ex-wife and access is being denied. It is essential to learn the details and to hear from both sides, if not directly, at least from their lawyers or court workers. Information such as threats of kidnapping, violent outbursts, fears of sexual abuse of the child, and arrears in child support payments is essential to your assessment and approach to the couple. On the other hand, occasionally one is faced with a male patient who has been denied access to his child by his ex-wife for no discernible reason. She will not accept his support payments because she does not want any contact whatsoever with her ex-husband. She may also project this feeling and attitude onto their child. Usually this woman has enormous unresolved rage at her ex-husband for leaving. She is totally incapable of separating her relationship with him from their child's relationship with him. Further, she tends to underestimate the father's importance to the emotional health of the child. Perhaps her own father-deprived background has left her with preconceived and distorted notions about the adequacy of divorced fathers. Key members of her family of origin may also reinforce these ideas and beliefs. Some of these women will respond to therapy; others will not or will refuse to see a therapist or mediator. The father's wishes are then best handled through family court.

Case Example 10

A family doctor requested an assessment of a couple in his practice who had recently separated. He was concerned about the reasons the mother of the children, aged 9, 7, and 5, was allowing the father only very scant and supervised access. He was worried about the father's mood and potential for retaliation against his wife. He was alarmed that the children were being deprived of an ongoing and loving relationship with their father.

Mr. and Mrs. J. came in together, and Mrs. J. began the interview by stating, "All of this silliness could be avoided if only Frank (Mr. J.) here could come to his senses, give up the tart he's been seeing, and come home where he belongs. And until he does, he will not see his children except under my supervision. They already see him as a scoundrel and a homebreaker." Since it appeared that Mrs. J. was coping with the complete shattering of her world and because she had had two previous depressions, therapy was allowed to proceed gently.

Individual visits enabled a sharper appreciation of each and of their stormy, chaotic 10-year marriage. Mr. J. was certain that the marriage was over and that he wished to remain separated. Mrs. J. normalized and denied any problems whatsoever in the marriage. She was becoming increasingly suspicious by the day and was coping less well at home with the children. She refused medication and refused to return. Over the phone she accused the therapist and her family doctor of siding with her husband against her: "You're both typical of this new wave of fathers who think they can bully their wives into handing over the children, regardless of their personal conduct." In response to her husband's petition in family court for more access, she fled that very evening with the children for Australia, her native country, from which she had emigrated 15 years earlier. Interestingly, she called the therapist from the airport to express her appreciation for his efforts. He urged her to reconsider her plans and to defer leaving her home so precipitously and impulsively, but this was to no avail. Five days later her father, a physician, telephoned to say that she was fine and so were the children. He was quite happy to have her home and away from his son-in-law "who I never liked anyway." He reiterated, "The children will be happy here, they will get on with their lives, and will forget their father in time."

Countertransference Issues

A common and complicating factor in many divorces is a third-party involvement with one of the spouses. In fact, it is not unusual for the partner who has another relationship to express ambivalence and regret, which is enhanced usually by the spouse's outrage and hurt, by the extended families' upset, and by society's disapproval. It is not easy for therapists either to remain neutral and effective in the face of very painful and intense emotions in the people they are trying to help. And for some therapists, the issue is too close to home, and they may not be able to treat the patient(s).

A man whose wife has become involved with a new man shortly before or after separation suffers a more profound sense of abandonment and intensified anger. He may have a subjective sense of being a "cuckold." Feelings of humiliation and retaliation are not unusual, and such men need to be watched closely for retributive violence and spiteful emotions contaminating visitation and custody deliberations. Previously, I have described a particular constellation of symptoms in two men whose wives had become involved with other women (14). These men, in addition to feelings of rejection and bewilderment, felt a blow to masculine self-esteem, assumed more than shared responsibility for the separation, totally blamed themselves, albeit transiently. They had difficulty appreciating the complex dynamics of this particular type of separation.

Case Example 11

Dr. K., a university professor, came to a therapist when he and his wife were about to separate. Mrs. K., a journalist, had fallen in love with another woman with whom she would be living immediately upon leaving her husband. Their 14-year-old son Mike would remain at home with his father and see his mother on weekends. On the surface all was quite civil.

Dr. K. was desperate. In his heart he was totally against the separation. He entreated the therapist to "try to talk some sense into her head—she doesn't know what she's doing—ruining Mike's life, my life, and ultimately her life." He went on, "Also, I don't believe she's really lesbian. I would call her a vulnerable neo-feminist who's a sitting duck for an aging lonely lesbian to get her hands on. It's all my fault, or mostly my fault. I know I've let her down by being so picky, so perfectionistic, and so absorbed in my work." Dr. K.'s statements about his wife alternated between professing undying love for her and demeaning mostly everything she had ever said or done.

Mrs. K. was seen alone. She was happy her husband had come to a therapist. She saw him as "really falling apart—I worry whether he'll make it on his own—Mike will help a lot." She was afraid of him; he had struck her twice and had made very frightening threats toward her and her partner Jane. She wondered about a restraining order but feared provoking him more for fear he would restrict visitation rights because of her lesbianism. She was quite clear about her own situation; indeed she had been unhappy in her marriage for a long time. She said

"I'm not exactly certain about Jane and me over the long term. At the moment I love her dearly and I'm experiencing something I've never ever felt before, anytime, in my life!"

Dr. K. worked alone for several months. Being in therapy helped to neutralize his rage and vindictiveness toward Mrs. K. and prevented him from acting it out. He also worked on underlying issues: his intellectualism, his profound need for control, his sexist notions about women, and his guilt about his marriage failing. Therapeutic support helped him to regain his shattered self-esteem and to begin to feel worthy again of someone's love and affection. He was seen with his son to address their adjustment to living together and also with Mrs. K. to discuss changes in access, his concerns about the boy's exposure to lesbianism, and her concerns about her husband having women sleep overnight and the impact of this on their son.

In addition to the abovementioned, the treatment of divorcing men includes some or all of the following tasks and goals: venting feelings (especially of anger, abandonment, hurt, failure, and guilt), regaining self-esteem (both social and sexual), understanding and working through problems of trust with women, reestablishing intimacy in new relationships, avoiding self-destructive behavior, enhancing fathering and co-parenting skills, and meeting and honoring financial and emotional responsibilities to children. Accepting and overcoming feelings of loneliness, enjoying one's own company, and learning to live alone are particularly difficult tasks for divorced men.

Transference Issues

Strong feelings of dependency on the therapist are not unusual in men in the middle of divorce. They will vary with the age of the patient, the age of the therapist, the sex of the therapist, and the degree of regression that has occurred in the man as a consequence of the divorce. In general, the more symptomatic difficulty the patient is having the more frightened and in need of the therapist's availability, strength, and comfort he will feel. This need will be greater if he is quite alone and does not have a supportive network of friends and family.

Male therapists must keep in mind the societal dictates in North America against men depending emotionally on other men (26). These forces may be at work in divorcing men who must defend very strongly against their feelings toward the therapist. For these men, recognizing and acknowledging strong and perhaps tender feelings for the therapist would make them feel very vulnerable, frightened, and "less a man." If one has taken a good history and has a working knowledge of the patient's object relations with other men, this type of transference can be anticipated and used therapeutically.

Another dynamic that may arise in the transference relationship is manipulation. Examples of this type of behavior are a) the patient bids the therapist to exert pressure on his reluctant wife to come in for marital or reconciliation therapy; b) the patient wants the therapist to communicate to his wife the details of his depressed mood, including perhaps his suicidal feelings and intent; and c) the patient attempts to enlist the therapist as an ally against his wife on issues ranging from defamation of her character and morals to custody contests. Whether to accede to or rebel against these demands is not the issue here for the therapist; identifying and working with the loss of control, sense of powerlessness, hurt pride, and desperateness of these divorcing men are the issue.

Patients who are borderline and those who are prepsychotic may develop intense transference jealousy, envy, and rage toward the therapist. This may be complicated by alcohol and drug abuse and may be characterized by frequent references to the therapist's marital status, children, or the state of the marriage itself. Assumptions and ideas about the therapist may be aired that are unfounded and perhaps quite distorted. Careful assessment of these statements, and the feeling state behind them, aids in diagnosing and revising drug treatment and psychotherapy.

Case Example 12

Mrs. L., a 42-year-old lawyer and father of three children, was quite depressed shortly after he and his wife separated. He was an acknowledged alcoholic, formerly with Alcoholics Anonymous, who had slipped back into drinking in the past six months. His wife, also a lawyer, precipitated the separation because she could no longer tolerate his drinking, his angry outbursts, and his verbal and physical abuse. They had been seeing another psychiatrist for marital therapy for about three months; once the decision to separate was made, they were not permitted to continue with the psychiatrist individually because "that was not his policy."

The assessment of Mr. L. was major depression complicated by alcohol abuse. He was quite symptomatic, with suicidal ideation but no plan. He agreed to an antidepressant and immediately returned to Alcoholics Anonymous. He was seen weekly, but there were one or two phone calls between visits. Initially he was friendly and rapidly became overfamiliar. Before calling the therapist, he had made some inquiries about his background and learned that they had attended the same university, at different times, and had been members of the same fraternity. He noted the pictures of the therapist's wife and children in the office and that stimulated a barrage of questions. He knew people who knew the therapist, including many other physicians in the city.

As their separation continued and it became clearer to Mr. L. that he and his wife would not be reconciling, he became angrier and angrier. He was angry at her, angry at the other psychiatrist for "not helping, and then bailing out," and angry at the therapist, whom he insulted one minute and apologized to the next. He said sarcastically "you have it all" and he had nothing. On one visit, he walked over and turned the picture face down. "I can't stand to look at them," he stated (the pictures were in fact not in his line of vision). He accused the therapist of smugness and lacking in sympathy, and taunted, "Your day will come; someday you'll be sitting in some shrink's office yourself with nothing to show for all your years of hard work."

What about competition in the male patient–male therapist dyad? This is most apt to occur with young, bright, achievement-oriented, and highly intellectualized patients working with male therapists who are about their own age. Review of their background often reveals a long history of competition with other men scholastically, athletically, and in the workplace. There may also be a prior history of "losing in love," that is, losing a girlfriend in adolescence or a woman friend in adult life to another man. The power disparity inherent in the therapeutic relationship is so formidable to these men that their characteristic defenses come into full force. It is essential that the therapist understand how much a "loser" this type of divorcing man feels inside and how much he may have to challenge and defeat the therapist in order to bolster his own self-worth.

Countertransference Issues for Male Therapists

Perhaps the commonest and most pervasive countertransference reaction when treating divorcing men is primal fear of one's own marriage and family life disintegrating. This fear can occur in married therapists of both sexes, but here we are interested in men working with men. A male therapist's own anxiety is apt to become heightened when a) he is in training and is not experienced in doing divorce work; b) the separation is wife-initiated and appears to occur "out of the blue" with no overt premorbid history of marital strain or unhappiness; c) the patient's age, personality, profession, and family situation are very similar to the therapist's; and d) both the patient and the therapist are struggling with life stage issues—especially mid-life.

During mid-life, all men are vulnerable and prone to periods of anxiety and uneasiness. Male psychiatrists, no matter how seasoned, how experienced in marital and divorce therapy, and how knowledgeable about themselves and their wives, cannot help but feel personally frightened as a consequence of therapeutic work with certain men in the midst of divorce. We see parts of ourselves in our male patients who leave their wives and who are left by their wives; we witness and share much of the terror and the agony, and sometime later, some of the joy and the happy times. There are parallels in other branches of medicine: Cardiologists fear chest pain, neurologists fear strokes, and oncologists fear sudden weight loss.

The unhappily married psychiatrist is inclined to feel countertransference envy toward divorcing men who are beginning to do well. He will resent their ability to come to terms with an unworkable marriage, to make a decision to separate, to enlist professional help, and to forge ahead with autonomy and self-interest. The subjective sense of feeling envious of a patient is always important and warrants honest introspection. Divorcing men who leave their marriages of 25 years for women 10 to 15 years younger may spark this type of reaction—which usually says much more about the therapist than the patient!

Specific countertransference feelings may arise in therapists treating men struggling with abandonment (14). Sex role rigidity may surface. Male therapists may overidentify and collude with the man's sense of outrage, indignation, and retribution. Insight building may be minimal, and adversariness in co-parenting may be aggravated. Female therapists may overnurture and overgratify dependency needs in these same men and not push enough self-sufficiency and independence. Both male and female therapists may have difficulty with very regressed men who are highly emotional, passive, and clinging. An unconscious sex bias that all men should be moderately strong and in control of their feelings causes these therapists to label this as "bad behavior" (for example, "he's acting like such a wimp!") rather than "symptomatic behavior."

Conclusion

In this chapter observations based on assessing and treating a large number of divorcing men, both in a private practice and in a hospital-based teaching setting, have been presented. These findings are impressionistic only. Much research is needed on psychiatric morbidity in men and divorce. This research needs to be longitudinal, prospective, comprehensive in scope, and controlled. Data obtained in this way will facilitate easier identification of men at risk, earlier intervention, and refinement of treatment approaches.

We cannot ignore the sociology of divorce in North America and the statistics: There are more than eight million women raising children under age 21 whose fathers do not live in the home (27) (U.S. Bureau of Census); one-third of them live below the poverty level; two-thirds of families entitled to child support collect no support at all; and fewer than 5 percent of all divorced, nonremarried women are entitled to receive alimony in a given year, and fewer still actually collect. This feminization of poverty has unwittingly been boosted by the legal system's reform in divorce policy away from the traditional adversarial system to non-fault divorce laws. Weitzman's 10-year study of no-fault divorce in California has concluded that the effect of the average divorce decree is to decrease the standard of living of the woman and any minor children in her household by 73 percent, while actually increasing that of the man by 42 percent (28).

These findings are shocking. Therapists cannot not be affected. They must incorporate this information into a better informed, penetrating, and balanced perspective when treating divorcing men.

References

1. National Center for Health Statistics: Births, marriages, divorces, and deaths for January, 1986. Monthly Vital Statistics Report (DHHS publication no. [PHS] 86-1120), April 21, 1986
2. Wallerstein JS, Kelly JB: The effects of parental divorce: experience of the preschool child. J Am Acad Child Psychiatry 14:600-616, 1975
3. Kelly JB, Wallerstein JS: The effects of parental divorce:

experiences of the child in early latency. Am J Ortho-psychiatry 46:20-32, 1976

4. Wallerstein JS, Kelly JB: The effects of parental divorce: experiences of the child in later latency. Am J Ortho-psychiatry 46:256-269, 1976
5. Shoettle UC, Cantwell DP: Children of divorce. J Am Acad Child Psychiatry 19:453-475, 1980
6. Wallerstein JS: Children of divorce: the psychological tasks of the child. Am J Orthopsychiatry 53:230-243, 1983
7. Brown P: Psychological distress and personal growth among women coping with marital dissolution. Dissertation Abstracts International 37:947-B, 1976
8. Brown P, Fox H: Sex differences in divorce, in Gender and Disordered Behavior: Sex Differences in Psychopathology. Edited by Gomberg ES, Franks V. New York, Brunner/Mazel, 1979
9. Wallerstein J: Women after divorce: preliminary report from a ten-year follow-up. Am J Orthopsychiatry 56:65-77, 1986
10. Hetherington ME, Cox M, Cox R: Divorced fathers. Family Coordinator 25:417-428, 1976
11. Jacobs JW: The effect of divorce on fathers: an overview of the literature. Am J Psychiatry 139:1235-1241, 1982
12. Jacobs JW: Treatment of divorcing fathers: social and psychotherapeutic considerations. Am J Psychiatry 140:1294-1299, 1983
13. Tepp AV: Divorced fathers: predictors of continued paternal involvement. Am J Psychiatry 140:1465-1469, 1983
14. Myers MF: Angry, abandoned husbands: assessment and treatment, in Marriage and Family Review. Edited by Sussman M. New York, Haworth Press, 1986
15. Gove W: The relationship between sex roles, marital status, and mental illness. Social Forces 51:238-244, 1972
16. Gove W: Sex, marital status, and mortality. American Journal of Sociology 79:45-67, 1973
17. Bloom BL: Changing Patterns of Psychiatric Care. New York, Human Sciences Press, 1975

18. Jacobs JW: Involuntary child absence problem: an affliction of divorcing fathers, in Divorce and Fatherhood: The Struggle for Parental Identity. Edited by Jacobs JW. Washington, DC, American Psychiatric Press, 1986
19. Friedman HJ: The father's parenting experience in divorce. Am J Psychiatry 137:1177-1182, 1980
20. Wallerstein JS, Kelly JB: Effects of divorce on the visiting father–child relationship. Am J Psychiatry 137:1534-1539, 1984
21. Myers MF: The abandoned husband. Medical Aspects of Human Sexuality 18:159-171, 1984
22. Weiss RS: Marital Separation. New York, Basic Books, 1975
23. American Psychiatric Association: Diagnostic and Statistical Manual of Mental Disorders (Third Edition, Revised). Washington, DC, American Psychiatric Association, 1987
24. Ross H, Sawhill I: Time of Transition: The Growth of Families Headed by Women. Washington, DC, Urban Institute, 1975
25. Levinson DJ: Seasons of a Man's Life. New York, Alfred A. Knopf, 1978
26. Pleck JH, Sawyer J: Men and Masculinity. Englewood Cliffs, NJ, Prentice-Hall, 1974
27. Takas M: Divorce: who gets the blame in "no fault"? Ms. Magazine, February 1986, p 48
28. Weitzman LJ: The Divorce Revolution: The Unexpected Social and Economic Consquences for Women and Children in America. New York, The Free Press, 1985

Chapter 4

Some Clinical Perceptions of Middle-Aged Divorcing Women

MARTHA KIRKPATRICK, M.D.

Some Clinical Perceptions of Middle-Aged Divorcing Women

*T*he change in divorce statistics is impressive, no matter which way you look at it, and there are a variety of ways to look at it. One way is to consider that there has been a 700 percent increase in divorce since 1900 (1). Another way to look at it is to compare the divorce rate relative to population of 1915, which was 1 divorce per 1,000 to that of 1966, which was 2.5 per 1,000, and 1979, which was 5.3 per 1,000 (2). (As of January 1986 the rate had dropped to 5.0 per 1,000 [3].) The statistics can also be viewed in terms of divorce rates to marriage rates. In 1976 there were 50 divorces for every 100 marriages (4). Oregon and California led the list with 83 and 89 divorces, respectively per 100 marriages. If this pattern continues, at least 50 percent of all women in their late 20s who are currently marrying will experience divorce; or of every 100 first marriages at least 50 will result in divorce. Twenty-nine of these women will remarry, thirteen of whom will divorce again.

Divorce has replaced death as the most likely cause of marital dissolution. According to a recent United States Census Report, more women in the United States today (ages 14 to 75) have had their first marriage end in divorce than in widowhood (4). In considering these statistics, however, it should be kept in mind that statistical record keeping is far better than it was earlier in this century, that segments of the population are included in the census that previously were ignored, that peo-

81

ple formalize their separation by legal divorce today, and that a greater percentage of the population marries today than earlier in the century.

The failure of marriage, with the shattered expectations and attendant miseries that precede divorce, is a psychological event. The divorce is a legal event. Yet the rules a society designs for the structure of divorce (who can divorce, for what reason, by what mechanism, and with what legal and social consequences to the individuals, their property, and their children) represent both the assumptions and values of that society and have profound psychological impact on its members. Divorce, like marriage, has been and continues to be very different for women than for men. The United States's War of Independence did endow "men" with "inalienable rights" and a governing power that derives its "just powers from the consent of the governed," but women were not so endowed. Women, in many ways (socially, economically, politically, and by internalized social mythology) remained in a feudal world. "A man's home is his castle" goes the old saying, and his wife remained a subject in his court. Not a revolution but a much slower evolution has worked toward the recognition of women as competent equal partners in all aspects of society. This evolution is manifest in the changes in the legal system's attitude toward women from The Married Woman's Property Acts in the mid-1800s to the no-fault divorce statutes in the 1970s.

In the 1800s divorce proceedings moved from state legislatures to civil courts. Cruelty and desertion were more readily considered grounds for divorce (5). This paralleled the growing idea of companionate marriage. Romance rather than property, money, or title has always been the accepted basis for choice of marriage partner in our country. Today we have, with the help of Hollywood and the mass media, reached the zenith in the expectation that romantic marriage not only is best, but will solve all problems and provide a life of endless joy.

At the same time, never has society had less to gain from the stable family and had so many impediments in its way. Families, once productive economic units, are now only units of consumption. From the point of view of an expanding economy, each broken family has doubled the consuming units, and the more units the better. Industry has discovered that single people are more committed to their careers, less resistant to move to a new site, less distracted by responsibilities at home, and so on.

The cost of raising children steadily increases. Children, like the family itself, no longer enhance a family's productivity, but only consume its resources. Marriage no longer joins families in an extended kinship with supportive rituals, but establishes a separate and often isolated new unit. With such a plethora of contradictory messages endowing marriage with unrealizable expectations on one hand and more complex and lonelier tasks than ever before on the other, it is no doubt that few have the resources to develop a workable marital partnership.

Blumstein and Schwartz (6) point out that the dramatic changes in marriages today are not the result of some sudden alteration in contemporary society. They suggest that the change began with the Industrial Revolution and the loss of the independence of the rural farm couple. The move to the city and the factory began the isolation of women from men and the productive world. A further impetus for change was World War II and the move of women into the work force. The significance of the domestic unit as the center of personal life and the source of satisfaction has been on the wane for some time.

Although the marriages of the younger generation are more likely to end in divorce than those of the older generation, there is an increase in divorce among persons of middle age and older. Only 4 percent of all divorces filed 30 years ago involved marriages of more than 15 years; the current figure is 25 percent, and about 16 percent involve couples who have been married 25 years or more. Since 1978, divorce has increased 50 percent for those between ages 40 and 65, and 35 percent for those over age 65 (6). Over the last several decades the highest percentages of divorces have occurred either between 5 to 9 years of marriage or after 15 years (7). Sociologists report that marital unhappiness peaks around the 20th year. It is greatest for women in their late 40s and early 50s, the same age period that sees the peak use of antidepressant drugs by women. It is women in this age range who are the most vulnerable to suffering from the consequences of the current divorce settlements.

Legal and Economic Consequences of Divorce

Although primarily concerned with the individual woman, her unique history, and her personal emotional distress, the clinician can be assisted by knowledge of current divorce experience in understanding the individual woman's plight and making a suitable evaluation. In the United States, socioeconomic decline following divorce is typically and uniquely a woman's experience. Weitzman, in a carefully documented appraisal of the consequences of California's 1970 no-fault divorce law, found that women experienced a 73 percent decline in their standard of living at the end of the first postdivorce year, whereas men experienced a 42 percent rise in their standard of living (8). Older women in long marriages from higher income levels ($40,000 annual income) experienced the greatest relative drop in standard of living.

No-fault divorce, now adopted in some form by every state except South Dakota, has recast the psychological context of the divorce process. It is no longer necessary for one spouse to accuse another of wrongdoing and impose on friends to perjure themselves as witnesses or hire detectives to procure evidence. There are no victims whose wrongs require legal redress. The framers of the law have succeeded in their aim of reducing the bitterness the previous adversarial process produced, but they were unprepared for the economic consequences for women. In redefining the rights and responsibilities of husbands and wives, they did not consider, according to Weitzman, that requiring proof of fault had long provided the one protection for economically dependent homemakers and some raising children. If a woman hadn't given her husband grounds for divorce, hadn't committed adultery or some other forbidden behavior, she had some leverage. She could agree to ask for the divorce herself on the grounds of the husband's behavior, but only if he first provided adequate support for her and the children. Without this leverage the resulting decline in support has been disastrous, especially for middle-aged homemakers.

The no-fault approach treats men and women as economic "equals at divorce, ignoring the economic inequality that marriage creates and the economic inequalities in the larger society" (8, p. xi). Even in two-career families, priority is usually given to the husband's career. The court does not treat the marriage as a partnership, and thus the husband's income is not "theirs" but his. More than 50 percent of older homemakers are denied alimony. The percentage is highest among low-income families. The amount of support on average amounts to the husband keeping two-thirds to three-fourths of the family income, while the wife and children together receive one-third.

By six months after divorce, 18 percent of those ordered to pay alimony are behind in their payments. For many older middle-class women this means a sudden drop from comfortable security to poverty. Even if they have worked at times during the marriage, their work histories are usually intermittent and without the intent of developing a career. Previous marketable skills have been lost and are probably obsolete. A woman's experience as homemaker and volunteer are not taken seriously in the job market, and the older woman is a pariah. Women in the job market earn 58 percent of men's earnings. Women account for 80 percent of those in the lowest paid occupations. Women who are able to take retraining courses after divorce do better, but this requires adequate alimony and support during the first few postdivorce years.

Property settlement is divided "equally" under no-fault law. Property includes tangible assets but not career assets, that is, salary, pension, medical insurance, education, business license, goodwill and credit in business, entitlement to company goods or services, or future earning power. In a divorce, a woman homemaker loses her job and the income and benefits that went with it while the husband loses only expenses. Often the house is sold in order to divide the assets. California, a community property state, divides tangible property 50/50. This means 50/50 for the two adults, yet 65 percent of divorcing couples have children, and 90 percent of children stay with the mother. Thus, at best, the mother and children have half of the property, the father the other half. In other states women and children together may receive less property than the father alone. Statutes do not recognize that mothers represent their children's as well as their own interests. Further, child care responsibilities limit a mother's employment. Although child support is awarded in 78 percent of divorce, it rarely covers half the cost of raising a child and stops when the child reaches the age of 18, just when college expense begins. In 1978 only 20 percent of fathers complied regularly with support orders, 15 percent complied irregularly, and 65 percent paid no support (9). Noncompliance was as true of high-income fathers as of low-income fathers.

One million children experience divorce each year in the United States. Most children of divorce live with mothers for at least five years after the divorce. Divorce has been said to result in "hardship, impoverishment and disillusionment for divorced women" (8, p. xii) and their children. This is the feminization of poverty. The single mother family is the fastest growing segment of the American poor. Children living in poverty rose from 14.9 percent in 1970 to 21.3 percent in 1982. Many previously comfortable women have been forced to apply for welfare and been further demoralized by finding this a demeaning experience (8). The 1981 Budget Reconciliation Act altered welfare policies disastrously for these women. Women were now forced to choose between inadequate welfare alone or inadequate wages alone (10).

Adding to this deplorable yet unacknowledged social disaster is the disturbing fact that mothers have been intimidated by threats of loss of custody despite having been primary care-takers (11). These threats kept mothers in bad marriages or were used to reduce support when divorce occurred. The court preference for joint custody has increased this threat. Chesler found that 70 percent of contesting fathers were awarded custody despite the fact that 87 percent had not been directly involved in child care and 67 percent had not even paid child support (11). Weitzman found that one-third of fathers were using custody threats for financial bargaining, while only 10 percent sought actual physical custody (8). Joint custody has further undermined the value of the work performed by the one who raises the child and the need for continuity of care. Joint custody persists as a threat to undermine the decisions of the caretaking parent.

The result of all this, Wallerstein found in a 10-year follow-up of 60 divorcing families, was continuing anger and bitterness among the women (12). Even remarriage did not mitigate the continuing sense of rage and betrayal. This was most marked in those middle-aged women who had been married for most of their adult lives. Wallerstein found these women over age 40 to have a much more difficult time reorganizing their lives and reestablishing social relationships: "At the ten-year mark many feel lonely and rejected, living in economic, social and psychological conditions well below that which they had achieved during their marriage" (12, p. 76). The potential for remarriage for women over age 44 compared to men is 56 to 100, respectively. A woman over 50 has only a 12 percent chance of remarriage (6, 13).

Despite the deplorable picture painted by these statistics, Wallerstein found some remarkable differences in the psychological effect of divorce on men and women (12). Divorce appeared to have resulted in a wide range of psychological changes and growth among women, but significantly less so among men. Although those who had not remarried complained of a loneliness not relieved by social and professional contacts, many had made major changes in psychological functioning: a striking rise in self-esteem, a new directness in acknowledging emotional needs and expressing feelings and thoughts, an increased capacity for humor, and a keenly realistic appraisal of self and the world. This was especially true for women who divorced in their 20s and 30s.

In Wallerstein's sample none of the women over age 40 had remarried; all had suffered a continuing decline in income with many worrying about meeting basic expenses. Loneliness approached 100 percent in these women. Psychosomatic symptoms were common, and 50 percent appeared clinically depressed. Nevertheless, these women had acquired much greater self-confidence and pride in their ability to take care of themselves and their children against great odds. Only one woman in the study would have opted for a return of the marriage and that was reluctantly. Most continued to feel intense anger and bitterness toward ex-husbands. Yet at the 10-year follow-up, 90 percent of the women and 70 percent of the men affirmed the divorce decision.

In Wallerstein's study, sex differences in regard to psychological change were striking. Sixty-four percent of the women improved in their psychological functioning, compared to only 16 percent of the men. Seventy-two percent of the men compared to sixteen percent of the women remained relatively unchanged. In only 10 percent of the couples had both partners benefited from the divorce. This appears to confirm Gove's finding that marriage was beneficial for men's mental health but dangerous for women's (14). Bernard reached a similar conclusion in *The Future of Marriage* (15). Divorce in spite of the unrecognized and unattended gross economic and social burdens can have a potentially positive effect on women's psychological development.

Psychological Consequences of Divorce

Despite the frequency of divorce, no one reaches this decision easily. In my clinical experience these decisions are rarely impulsive. A long period of denial, ambivalence, guilt, and fearful expectations of the future precedes the decision to divorce, especially in middle-aged women. Middle-aged women who are divorced by their husbands, often with little or no preparation, face an even greater sense of loss and betrayal, which requires extraordinary inner resources to surmount. For women, socialized to define themselves by their relationship to others, the shift from wife to nonwife can amount to a loss of identity, a shift to nonperson. The therapist can help in relieving internal inhibitions against the development of other sources of self-esteem and gratification and in supporting a more autonomous sense of self. After divorce, the middle-aged woman who was prepared for the life of an auxiliary is expected by a social and judicial system in transition to become a self-initiating, independent competitor in the economic jungle. Society has prepared no bridge, no refuge for these women caught in the transition. They may be only marginally able to compensate for the loss, even with the best therapeutic effort.

Case Example 1

A woman in her mid-40s was referred by her internist. She had discovered that her husband's prolonged business trips had been to the beach apartment of a younger woman colleague. Their marriage of 20 years had seemed relatively successful. She had graduated from college with a degree in history and had held various clerical jobs early in the marriage, but had not worked since her children were born. Her husband's career had prospered, requiring a number of moves to other countries and other cities. In the recent moves she had been able to remodel the current house so that the family had financially benefited from the sale. She was also actively involved in developing a social life for her husband with his colleagues. One child was still living at home.

Five years before, during another period of her husband's prolonged absences she had had an affair with a neighbor. Although their sexual contact was rare, the relationship had provided an intimacy, concern, and gentleness she had not known before. She had felt extremely guilty, although she was aware of the marriage's deficiencies and her husband's occasional peccadillos. She had concluded the affair after a few months, feeling that the marriage was her first priority. This affair remains a bittersweet memory of renunciation.

When confronted with his behavior, her husband declared that he was indeed seriously involved with someone else and had been planning to divorce her. He moved out the next week. She went through a period of shock and disbelief, followed by alternate rage, helplessness, and despair. The pain dealing with the children and the humiliation of telling friends and family was exhausting. She threw herself into a training program for historical renovation. This was compromised by periods of clinical depression with severe insomnia, weight loss, apathy, and suicidal ideation. She reviewed her early life, her many disappointments with an adored but remote father who had died early in her marriage. She saw elements of her efforts to interest and please her father in her relationship with her elusive husband. Being good had provided the only possible hope of being loved and protected. Now it was clear that "being good" was not to be rewarded. By the end of her training program she had regained some sense of personal worth but remained lonely, fragile, and with a deep sense of betrayal and wasted sacrifices.

Women seem caught in a socialization process that requires the inhibition of personal ambition, even of personal development, in order to fit the role of the nurturing auxiliary in marriage. Blumstein and Schwartz discovered that marriages were likely to dissolve if the husband perceived his wife as committed to her work or ambitions (6). In fact, educated women with a capacity for higher earnings had a four times greater likelihood of divorce (and a greater likelihood of remaining single after divorce).

Blumstein and Schwartz also noted that the old notion of women staying in marriages not out of satisfaction with their lot but because they do not have the resources to support themselves still retains a great deal of truth to it. Yet even for those women who do have the necessary earning power, reaching the decision to leave an inhibiting or debilitating marriage is difficult.

The Stages of Divorce

Stage 1: The Planning Stage

The acceptance of divorce as a legitimate solution to an unsatisfactory marriage, despite its current frequency, can take a very long time—sometimes many, many years. Socialization as a caretaker, a displaced desire to please the father and fulfill his (or the patriarchal society's) myth of femininity, and/or guilt and fear over angry impulses all play a part in creating chronic depression or undermining the woman's efforts to take action in her own behalf.

Case Example 2

A 45-year-old nurse practitioner with two teenage children came to therapy stating she had been contemplating divorce for 10 years. Her husband was subject to sullen rages and was otherwise withdrawn; he rarely participated in family life. The children were frightened of him, as were many of the patient's friends. The patient had had several long extramarital affairs that had been sexually satisfying, but she found herself unable to remain in love. She would lose respect for the lover and begin to devalue him, resulting in the feeling that she was incapable of love and that she deserved to be with a man like her husband. She was the only child of ardent pacifists who regarded any expression of displeasure as dangerous. Her husband carried the burden of being angry for both, while she nursed the sick world. In other relationships any experience of disappointment or anger was quickly repressed, but the object was demoted to insignificance to avoid the risk of a recurrence of hurt and hostile feelings. Once able to tolerate and make use of her own angry feelings, she could complete and carry out plans for a long-overdue divorce. She has recently remarried.

The inhibiting of aggression in the service of self-development so often promoted by women's early experience can interfere not only with career development, but with the very nurturing skills this inhibition was meant to enhance. Arendell and Wallerstein (10, 12) found mothers describing improved relationships with children following divorce, despite the hardships and the tensions around custody and support.

Case Example 3

An obstetrician referred a 37-year-old married woman for what was described as a postpartum depression following the birth of her third child. There were no vegetative signs and no evidence of psychotic process. She spoke in a soft voice, often through tears, about her sense of weakness and demoralization. Her career as an executive in a public relations firm seemed doomed due to her lack of confidence and her submissiveness. Although a dream early in therapy suggested dissatisfaction with her marriage, consciously she was only grateful to her accountant husband for his patience and support during this depressed period.

It became evident that the depression was longstanding but had deepened currently because of guilt over wanting to be more involved with the third child, a girl, than she had been with her first two. She felt required to return to full-time work as soon as possible. The conflict around leaving her little girl revived experiences of loss and deprivation with her own depressed and emotionally flat mother. As a child she had turned to her father, a businessman enthusiastically engrossed in his work and his hobbies. Her efforts to please him had led to her own professional career and ultimately her choice of husband. She had seen herself as a defective child, dependent on her father's, and then her husband's, wisdom and competence. Both required that she work hard and be obedient.

As this emerged in therapy, she was able to limit her professional work to part-time and was able to increasingly enjoy her children. She developed a closer and more confiding relationship with her mother, who at the patient's suggestion, began seeing a therapist for her own lifelong depression. The patient developed new social and technical skills that she put to use in her agency. As her social relationships broadened, she discovered her often bossy husband was really quite timid and relied on her to create their social life. As her self-esteem increased she returned to hobbies she had given up when she married. She became increasingly aware of the marked differences between her husband and herself in regard to interests, life-style, and hopes for the future. Her husband was committed to rising rapidly in his career and was rarely available for family experiences. She longed for a life devoted to the outdoors in a small community. Her sense of competence and adequacy as a woman increased, and she felt less frightened of and dependent on the approval of father and husband. After three years of planning to divorce and one year of separation, she was able to initiate a divorce action. She returned to her career with new enthusiasm and confidence, but has found ways of continuing the greater intimacy with her children.

Stage 2: The Divorce Process

Once the plan to divorce has been accepted, the process stage begins. Regularly in my practice, no matter what the marriage experience has been, no matter how fearful the expectations of punishment, no matter who initiates the divorce or why, the woman begins by announcing she is lucky that her husband is an honest and responsible provider and will not cheat his family of adequate support. Often this idealization of the husband as provider leads her to accept one lawyer (usually his) who will draw up the agreement, or she may simply take no steps to find legal counsel, since the husband can be counted on to provide and protect. Evidence of this husbandly trait is often not forthcoming. Spousal support is awarded in less than 14 percent of all divorces and received in less than 7 percent. So it is not surprising that over half of all poor families are female headed and over one-third of female headed families are below the poverty line (10).

Case Example 4

A 35-year-old teacher with a 10-year-old child reported increasing anxiety and depression around violent battles with her husband of 12 years. She experienced physical beatings one to three times a year and had been locked out of the house on several occasions. She held herself responsible for these attacks because she "yelled back," and she felt reprehensible for not enjoying her husband's impulsive and rather violent sexual overtures.

Although she contributed significantly to the family income, her husband had always managed the family's finances on his own. After many trial separations, several years of couple therapy, and several trial reunions, the divorce process began. Her husband prepared a financial settlement. She struggled against the discovery that her husband was protecting his interests and that she would have to protect her own. She discounted the therapist's efforts as overzealous feminism. She transferred to a male therapist in the hope he could protect her image of her husband as provider. He did not, and the divorce is slowly proceeding.

Case Example 5

A 48-year-old mother of three children in their late teens came to therapy because of depression. She had suffered from an acute reactive depression after the birth of her last child. At that time she felt torn between a successful career of her own and the demands of her family and her husband's career. Her depression abated with therapy over the next year and she devoted herself to her children and her husband's professional development, always fearing a return of the depression. Her husband was gone for extended periods, during which the family relaxed, only to be galvanized into a frenzy of preparations in an effort to avoid his critical scrutiny on his return. But some error was always found.

He was sensitive, hypochondriacal, meticulous, exacting, and very needy of his family's constant admiration and attention. Rare sexual contact was strained and unsatisfying. The patient felt drained, longed for an opportunity to realize her own ambitions before it was too late, and was haunted by the conviction that she was too weak, too vulnerable to depression to consider separation. As she entered therapy, her children were moving into their own lives. She saw herself as a collection of functions surrounding her husband. Efforts to pursue a separate career were repeatedly interrupted or overshadowed by her husband's career.

After a trial separation, the divorce process began with the patient claiming that she need not worry about money. She resisted seeking legal advice, resisted the legal advice she eventually received anyway, and clung to the belief that she simply couldn't understand figures, rather than understand that her highly successful husband meant to minimize financial support.

Stage 3: The Aftermath

The rupture of the idealization of the husband as protector and provider leads to a sense of betrayal and rage. A secret pact is revealed in which trust and fiscal innocence are maintained by the wife in return for being protected and provided for. This pact predates the marriage, though the marriage may have been based on it. The discovery that she must not only provide for herself, but must protect herself from his exploiting her economic dependence on him, although embittering, is often also liberating. The requirement to trust and be innocent is suspended. Despite the anger and lowered standard of living, some divorcing women, especially those who have delayed action for many years, are caught up in a euphoria. This can be a dangerous state in which investments of money and emotion may be made impulsively, at times reflecting a continuing effort to idealize the protective role of a new and better man. This idealization, while encouraged by socialization and romanticized by literature, contains important residues of incomplete separation/individuation. This process may have been inhibited in early life by the fear that autonomy would sever the emotional and social ties so instrumental in female development.

The euphoria may also represent a manic defense against losses, fears of the future, and depression. However, the sense of release can represent a new hope, an opportunity for growth, a chance to finally proceed with delayed separation/individuation and individualization. The economic losses for divorcing women have been reported here, but these are not the only losses. Changes of domicile, neighborhood, schools, and extracurricular activities add to the disruption for both divorcing women and their children. These problems put enormous strain on the women's emotional resources, adaptive capacities, and parenting skills.

In my experience, however, the most painful discovery for the divorcing woman is the loss of her social support system. Middle-aged women who have been part of the married world for many years are unaware that this world is chauvinistic, elitist, and highly ritualized around the existence of a husband. Divorcing women are shocked and embittered over the loss of friends, activities, and emotional support they had assumed belonged to them rather than to their marital status. The change in economic circumstances, the necessity to go to work, usually full-time, and the loss of membership in various clubs and/or volunteer activities destroy the paths of interaction with old friends.

Case Example 6

A 52-year-old housewife divorcing after 26 years of marriage to a successful television personality was distressed to find friends failing to return her calls. The couple had lived for extended periods of time on both coasts and had long-time friends in both cities. Old friends were occasionally free for lunch, but no longer invited her to dinner parties or to share evening concert tickets. She blamed this on West Coast superficiality and returned to the East where "tradition and true friendship were respected." She was deeply hurt to find her friends graciously indifferent to her need for closeness and support, while she heard of her husband's presence at parties with these same old friends. Building new networks was a painful and only partially successful process for her.

Women who are involved in the work world prior to divorce have a network of support separate from marital status, similar to the husband's career network. This is enormously valuable as a source of social sustenance and a bridge to new social networks. The middle-aged woman who is faced with a loss of social support systems and the necessity to find employment may need the therapist's active intervention to direct her to community resources where new networks can be established. Although the stigma of divorce has decreased and the employment and educational possibilities for women have increased, the consequences of economic and social loss pose a social problem yet to be addressed by social planning agencies (10).

Remarkably enough, despite the losses, struggles, and burdens imposed by divorce, in my experience few of the women who have initiated and concluded a divorce claim to regret it. They regret the loss of financial security, the loss of a higher standard of living, and the loss of sexual companionship. Yet by the end of two years many report an increasing reliance on their own capacities and judgment, a discovery of inner resources, and a sense of self-esteem that is not derived from an attachment to another. Many report improved relationships with children, a revitalization of relationships with kin, and, most particularly, an increasing pride in themselves.

For the middle-aged divorced woman, remarriage seems the only possibility to restore the lost standard of living and sense of financial security. Although it is unlikely for women of this age, many resist it when it is available. Blumstein and Schwartz in their study of cohabiting couples found women who had previously been married less likely to hope the relationship would lead to marriage than similar women who had not previously been married. This was not true of cohabiting men.

Conclusion

The gradual but all-encompassing changes in society since the Industrial Revolution, the massive increase in population, and the complexities of contemporary life have changed the couple and the family forever. The marriage contract, legal and psychological, no longer works, especially for women. The experiments with new styles of relating are painful and inconclusive. For those caught in the transition, it is costly, often tragic. New contracts that protect children are clearly essential. Perhaps the efforts of lesbians and gay men to create contracts for the care of children conceived outside of marriage will provide a useful guide to heterosexuals as well (16).

The last 100 years have seen the development of increasingly smaller social units. The "nuclear family" is good for the consumer market but places enormous strains on the marital couple, who are the major source of each other's need for adult affiliation and support. This is even more burdensome because of the incredible mobility of the American family, which causes social ties outside the home to be repeatedly ruptured. Women's characteristic strong need for social affiliation makes these ruptures especially painful for them and may reveal or overburden a marginally supportive marriage. Whatever the causes, divorce is an increasingly common experience in women's lives. Whether divorce becomes an opportunity for growth in the midst of losses and changes or an embittering devastation of life's expectations depends in part on the therapist's understanding of the complex balance of losses and gains and of the personal inhibitions to the tasks of separation/individuation.

References

1. Zwerling I: The Struggle for Survival: A Psychiatrist's Perspective on the Contemporary Family in America (Symposium). Smith, Kline and French Co., June 1978
2. Norton AJ; Glick PC: Marital instability in America: past, present and future, in Divorce and Separation: Context, Causes, and Consequences. Edited by Levinger G, Moles OC. New York, Basic Books, 1979
3. National Center for Health Statistics: Births, marriages, divorces, and deaths for January, 1986. Monthly Vital Statistics Report (DHHS Pub. No. [PHS] 86-1120), April 21, 1986
4. Statistical Abstract of the United States. Washington, DC, U.S. Government Printing Office, 1978
5. Basch N: The emerging legal history of women in the United States: property, divorce, and the Constitution. Signs: Journal of Women in Culture and Society 12(1):97-117, 1986

6. Blumstein P, Schwartz P: American Couples. New York, William Morrow, 1983
7. Bane M: The American divorce rate: what does it mean? what should we worry about? in The Challenge of Change. Edited by Horner M, Nadelson C, Notman M. New York, Plenum Press, 1983
8. Weitzman L: The Divorce Revolution. New York, Free Press, 1985
9. U.S. Department of Commerce, Bureau of the Census: Child Support and Alimony 1978. Washington, DC, U.S. Government Printing Office, 1981
10. Arendell T: Divorce: a woman's issue. Feminist Issues 4:41-61, 1984
11. Chesler P: Mothers on Trial: The Battle for Children and Custody. New York, McGraw-Hill, 1985
12. Wallerstein J: Women after divorce: preliminary report from a ten year follow-up. Am J Orthopsychiatry 56:65-77, 1986
13. Luria Z, Meade R: Sexuality and the middle-aged woman, in Women and Midlife. Edited by Baruch G, Brooks-Gunn J. New York, Plenum Press, 1984
14. Gove W: The relationship between sex roles, marital status and mental illness, in Beyond Sex Role Stereotypes: Readings Toward a Psychology of Androgyny. Edited by Kaplan A, Bean J. Boston, Little, Brown, 1976, pp. 281–292
15. Bernard J: The Future of Marriage. New York, World Press, 1972
16. Pies C: Considering Parenthood: A Workbook for Lesbians. San Francisco, Spinsters Inc., 1985

Chapter 5

Sexual Behavior of Women After Divorce

JUDITH H. GOLD, M.D., F.R.C.P.(C)
CAROL C. NADELSON, M.D.

Chapter 5

Sexual Behavior of Women After Divorce

Sexuality is simply not biology. . . . Sexuality involves a capacity to trust and feel trustworthy, to be intimate and separate without intolerable anxiety (1).

Identity and Intimacy

Marriage usually begins with a spoken commitment between partners and an unspoken assumption of intimacy, faithfulness, and mutual caring and respect. Sometimes a partner's inability to live up to these expectations is repressed, denied, or simply not questioned. As has been stated in previous chapters, many factors can contribute to the erosion of trust and intimacy, including belittling, opposing views of gender roles, and the individual psychosocial growth and development of each partner, which may move along different paths.

That all of these are important and can have potentially destructive consequences can be seen by the high divorce rate in North America, where one in two first marriages end in divorce. The effects of marital dissolution are discussed in other chapters of this monograph; the focus of this chapter is on the sexual aspects of women's adjustment to the ending of the marriage.

The growth of the capacity for intimacy is gradual, beginning with the establishment of what Erikson called "basic trust" in infancy (2). The individual comes to accept that caring can be constant and reliable, rather than hurtful and capricious. As we grow through childhood we establish not only a gender identity but also a sexual self-concept (3). This plays a part in our formation of personal identity during adolescence, always influenced by our ability to trust.

The capacity for intimacy depends on many factors, including one's identity, the concept of one's self. The quality of a relationship is determined by each partner's identity as well as by the need for, and the ability to tolerate, intimacy. Here role expectations are also very important, and these are determined by sociocultural factors, as well as by each individual's needs and all the aspects of his or her identity. As discussed earlier, marriage can have severe effects upon each partner's identity and upon the ways in which a person learns to interrelate with others. If a marriage has been acrimonious, abusive, or intimidating, or if it has been filled with conflict, deceit, or disrespect, it is likely to leave a legacy of insecurity and to challenge a woman's self-esteem and even her identity. This may make it difficult for her to form new attachments or to tolerate or trust men.

Intimacy After Divorce

Following a marital breakdown, many women turn to others for support (4). Such social supports are recognized as buffers for stress (5). They may also encourage the sustenance of angry and unpleasant feelings, particularly if the woman uses others to confirm her own reactions and is not able to explore her feelings in greater depth. Anger and lack of trust against the former spouse can remain undiminished and can generalize and transfer to other men.

Thus many women initially after a divorce state that they cannot imagine being interested in a man again, even just for a casual "date." This need to remain separate from another person is part of the process of reintegration of the self, of reestablishing trust in one's self and beginning to regain a tolerance of intimacy. Many women comment that they cannot bear the thought of getting to know someone else and having that person know them. They feel vulnerable and mistrustful, especially when they have been rejected by someone to whom they revealed themselves. Their anger is often displaced onto others.

The length of time it takes for these feelings to dissipate is related to self-esteem and to the prior depth of existing trust in others. Narcissistic injury is modified by ego strengths that can be weakened by the quality of the relationship within the marriage. A constant hammering at self-esteem by a denigrating spouse requires much ego strength to be sustained. When sexual relations have also been poor, many women doubt their sexual attractiveness and their ability to enjoy sex.

Case Example 1

J.T. had been married for 22 years when her husband announced he was leaving the home and the marriage. He stated that he was unhappy with her and that he needed to live apart in order to sort out his own wants and goals. Initially J.T. was stunned by this decision and unwilling to believe it. She felt overwhelmed and unable to make any decisions or to be alone. Reviewing their marriage, she recalled the jobs she had taken only in order to support them while he studied and the jobs she had refused in order to stay in a city where his career could be furthered. J.T. felt she had been forced to make most of the daily household and parenting decisions because her husband was rarely willing to do so. He would then criticize whatever she had concluded.

Furthermore, he constantly made light of her work and its importance. Their sexual relationship had been poor since he had been disinterested increasingly over the past few years. After he left she felt discarded, unattractive, and fearful. All of these feelings escalated enormously when she discovered he had been involved with a woman friend of theirs for at least two years before leaving the marriage. Friends rallied around to offer her support, and she gratefully accepted their help and sympathetic listening. However, some were also friendly to the husband and passed on her statements to him. She again felt betrayed and withdrew from all of them. For several months she avoided all social interactions other than at her job or with her sisters and children.

About six months after the marriage had broken down, J.T. went on a trip related to her employment. While at this conference she met an old colleague and they spent an evening talking enjoyably. She felt close to this man and to her surprise found herself sexually involved with him that night. She returned home feeling more confident of herself as a woman and more willing to examine the possibility of future relationships. This growth of self-esteem began to extend into her job, and she became slowly more certain of her abilities. She made some tentative steps to establish new friendships outside their previous circle of friends. Nevertheless, J.T. remained convinced she would not allow herself to become attached to any man, feeling she could never trust again.

Sexuality After Divorce

Some women seek one or more casual sexual encounters to reinforce their esteem and their belief that they are attractive and have the desire and capacity to enjoy sex. Many women fear they are sexually inadequate or damaged and are afraid to attempt a long-term relationship again. Anger also plays a role, in that a woman may unconsciously or at times deliberately seek to hurt the spouse who rejected her by demonstrating her attractiveness to others.

Case Example 2

B.K., age 32, left her husband after 12 years of marriage. They had married while in college, and she had continued to work after the birth of their child four years later. His job involved a great deal of travel, during which he was unfaithful frequently and openly. He expected her to accept his behavior, which he viewed as natural during separations. When at home he wanted her to share his varied sexual interests. She felt increasingly unattractive and without libido in the marriage. B.K. decided to study further in an attempt to bolster her self-esteem. While doing so she met several men who found her very appealing and had a series of brief affairs whenever her husband was away. Initially she was conscious of her anger and wish for revenge; later she enjoyed the relationships themselves. At this point she decided to leave the marriage and find a more mutually satisfying and acceptable mate.

It is not uncommon for divorcing spouses to find themselves together for a night or a weekend. Attracted to each other again by some positive aspects of their marriage and by dependency needs, they feel a resurgence of sexual feelings. These encounters may occur several times during the divorce process. Often enjoyable, sexual relations may be all that remains between them. This can be confusing for one or both of them, especially if the episode dissolves into their customary arguments and distancing. For many couples such sexual intimacy is part of the work of separation and the regaining of autonomy for each. However, for the woman whose self-esteem is low and who felt abused within the marriage, such occurrences can add to feelings of being manipulated, weak, and dependent. She may feel helpless to resist her ex-husband, feeling needy of caring and sexual satisfaction, and may denigrate herself for this. For others, such relations are a comfortable outlet for physical needs without the risks involved in forming a new liaison.

In other cases, early in the separation the woman finds herself attracted to another male. They become involved and intimate quickly, often cohabiting although not always marrying. Without resolving the conflicts from the first relationship, she regains self-esteem from a new dependency and from demonstrating to her husband that another man cares for her. However, her ego strengths remain unchanged so she is vulnerable to a repetition of the marriage. This formation of an early new alliance is discussed in more detail in Chapters 1 and 2, but the following brief case example is illustrative.

Case Example 3

C.D., age 33, finally asked her husband to leave after 10 years of marriage during which he had abused her physically and psychologically. His violence continued during the divorce process and battle for custody of their children. She turned to her women friends for emotional support during this period and was introduced to a man who was also divorcing. They quickly became dependent on each other and drew strength from their interactions. Although they maintained separate residences, their sexual relationship restored her feelings of attractiveness. Her former spouse threatened harm to this man should they meet. This new relationship continued for five years, during which C.D. made every effort to be receptive to this man's needs while making her own secondary. She became aware gradually that she was as dissatisfied and feeling as psychologically abused as before. She began to separate from him, painfully.

For other women the wish to avoid relationships with men continues, and women friends are seen as confidantes and supporters. Historically, women on their own have turned to other women for the social and emotional support they need to continue on with their lives or move toward new goals. In the last century, as women were educated and developed careers outside of the home, they often lived together. This was an accepted tradition. These relationships were often loving and intimate (6). Many married women also found the emotional intimacy they required only in friendships with another woman or groups of women friends. Some of these friendships became sexual. This continues to be a pattern of adaptation; the previously heterosexual woman finds acceptance and tolerable intimacy with women. Some, however, become involved in such an intimate relationship at the same time they are beginning involvements with men.

Homosexuality After Divorce

The arousal of homosexual feelings is confusing and unacceptable for many women. Sexuality may be only one aspect of their homosexual involvement. They may also seek satisfaction of dependency needs, a sympathetic ear to descriptions of the hurt and fury engendered by the marriage and the divorce, or an unthreatening, loving, and supportive relationship (often the first such relationship) (7). The woman thus becomes sister, mother, and lover, a combination difficult to withdraw from.

Yet, prior sexual identity conflicts with this new love, and the woman may be unsure of herself and her new identity.

For other women their relationship is an acknowledgment of previously repressed homosexual desires. Marriage may have served to reinforce the repression, as had the numerous struggles and crises within the marriage. Societal and parenting roles as well as religious prohibitions against lesbianism also are important constraints that may have served to prevent the expression of these feelings (8).

Earlier in this book we discussed the development of gender-related roles in our society. The previous chapters have described the various aspects of psychosexual development in men and women, and how development is affected by divorce. A woman who has felt herself diminished in comparison to a man, and who has not felt her intimate needs to have been appreciated or reciprocated, often finds the equality and acceptance she has longed for in a new loving relationship with a woman.

Social conditioning and internal confusion may prevent her from mentioning the quality of the involvement to others, even to her psychotherapist. She may choose to go into therapy in an attempt to resolve the conflicts aroused within her by this new relationship, but may present with other symptoms.

In other instances, the love of another woman becomes restorative of ego-strength, and the divorced woman's self-esteem rises. She may then leave the relationship, or its sexual portion, and return to new heterosexual beginnings. Some women find all the support, love, and sexual satisfaction they need in their new homosexual relationships and continue this lifestyle. However, for other women social interactions remain difficult even within the safety of an ego-acceptable lesbian pairing. These women often have not been able to work through their lack of trust. The same problems arise with sharing, intimacy, and communication that had occurred within the marriage. In these cases, it may be that the woman has chosen a woman lover who has the same overwhelming, but desired, traits of the former husband in order to satisfy her needs.

The greater sensitivity to her that this woman displayed may have helped her deny this initially.

Finally, just as there are men who are able to detect and respond to the unconscious needs of a newly divorced woman, there are also waiting female seducers. Unlike in the previous examples where two women become lovers through friendship, whether one has previously acknowledged herself to be lesbian or not, there are women who deliberately set out to seduce the new divorcée. The relationship may go well, of course, depending on the true depth of commitment.

Case Example 4

W.A., a 40-year-old woman, left her marriage after years of enduring her husband's rages and physical abuse. Following a bitter court case, she won custody of their young daughter. Throughout the divorce and custody battle she was strongly supported by an older woman who became her lover. This woman left a lesbian relationship of many years as their involvement grew from friendship and sympathy into intimacy and finally sexuality.

W.A. was able to acknowledge her previously repressed homosexuality, and the two lived together for several years. During this time W.A. gradually became discomforted by her partner's frequently violent anger toward her and by her increasing perception of herself as subservient within the dyad.

She then met another woman who was trying to leave a similar lesbian relationship. The two women offered each other great support and a mutually quiet respect that both found ego rewarding. They began living together, and W.A. felt equal to another for the first time.

Three years later she sought treatment for acute anxiety and depression of some months duration. She stated that she felt misunderstood and neglected by her mate, that they argued constantly, and that she would leave except for their financial interdependence. She had left her job about two years before and had started a postgraduate course, just as her lover had begun a new business. She had not discussed this change but had implemented and then announced it. As a result, the couple had been in financial difficulties ever since and gradually communicated even less. They became enraged with each other and neither knew how to express her anger or how to reach out to the other without fearing loss of self.

The third relationship brought W.A.'s difficulties of trust and intimacy into sharp focus and she was finally able to seek help to change. The caring and equality of the initial phase of this latter relationship allowed her insight into her own psychological problems and helped her begin the process of change.

Case Example 5

F.B., a 45-year-old woman, had recently separated from her husband of 25 years, although they still shared the same house. She was unable to leave because of his physical disabilities. In addition, they had the same profession and worked in partnership. Their two children had already left home.

Throughout the marriage, F.B. had been the strong partner and had supported her husband through years of study and pecuniary problems. She had then taken professional education herself. In the last years of the marriage she began to feel imposed upon and angry. She relied on a few close women friends for support and ventilation. She became involved in a feminist political group where she met several women who were lesbian and began to examine her own sexuality.

She acknowledged her own homosexual feelings, but was reluctant to become involved in such a relationship because of her community position and her expectation of her childrens' reactions. On a visit to a friend in another city she found herself intensely sexually involved with this woman. The experience allowed her to admit her own sexual feelings to herself.

Then she began to deal with her ambivalence toward her husband, which had been a mixture of guilt and anger. She began to confront the guilt-producing interactions with him and learn to assert herself more effectively. She was then able to leave the marriage. She maintained close friendships with several women and hoped to find a lover.

In F.B.'s case, the marriage breakdown brought her into contact with supportive friends and enabled her to acknowledge her own sexual orientation. In addition, she learned self-assertion and freed herself from repetitive behaviors induced by guilt.

Case Example 6

N.C., a 46-year-old woman, was divorcing from her husband of over 25 years. She was experiencing anxiety that at times overwhelmed her, and she frequently became angry and wanted to hurt herself. One of two sisters, she had been raised by strict parents who taught her from early childhood never to express anger. She was brought up to be dutiful to her parents, family, and later to her husband. She married her university boyfriend just as they graduated. They had three children over an eight-year period.

N.C.'s husband was frequently unable to go to work and she always made excuses for him. His job involved community relations in their small town. She began to participate in some of the same activities. However, she felt her first obligation was at home. She always attempted to follow his wishes and rarely spoke her own thoughts. Despite her shyness she became active in a few volunteer groups and soon was sought out by others for her confidence and empathy. Her husband tried to discourage these activities, and as she became more successful at them he grew increasingly angry.

He was then transferred to a larger town, where she was asked to resume these volunteer jobs. She did, over his strong objection, but continued to devote herself primarily to their home and family. She was unable to discuss her feelings with him because she felt intimidated and would cry. Finally she left home precipitously when her husband was in a rage and she feared that he might beat her.

After a few months, N.C. began seeing an old male friend whose marriage had also just dissolved. She enjoyed the chance to share feelings with another person and was pleased to discover herself as a sexual being. However, over the next year this relationship petered out. Her husband meanwhile wanted to remarry and began pressing for a divorce and property settlement. He argued over support for the children and over every item in their home. She became increasingly anxious and indecisive. She leaned heavily on a few women friends for support and advice. One of these women was especially understanding and available to her. She felt increasingly close to her and realized she loved her and wanted a sexual relationship with this woman.

The friend clearly stated that she was heterosexual and happily married but was very willing to remain her good friend and to support her. N.C. was initially shocked at her own feelings but came to terms with her ability to love another woman, while resenting this woman's unavailability. They remained close friends. Meanwhile N.C. relied on a woman lawyer to help her through her legal proceedings. She began to confront her own anger at her husband, to recognize its legitimacy, and to try to express it through appropriate self-assertion.

N.C.'s case demonstrates the effect of social values and attitudes about women's roles on a person's psychosocial development. She described her upbringing as "Victorian" and struggled with the guilt that colored and controlled all her reactions. Her community work allowed her to develop some self-esteem and gave her an indication of her own strength. This frightened her husband, who used anger to control her. Her first relationship after the separation revealed feelings to her that she had repressed totally and gave her enough ego strength to continue. In her women friends she found the intimacy, trust, and warmth she had longed for—for many years unknowingly longed for—and then desired a total involvement with a woman. The caring and support of several other friends —all women—sustained her as she battled to learn about herself and to live with herself.

Case Example 7

L.D., age 35, was hospitalized by her family physician for multiple somatic complaints. She and her husband lived together, but she had moved to another bedroom about a year before. She described her husband as supportive, accepting, quiet, and responsible and felt guilty that she had no interest in him. Married for about 15 years, they had no children and she had been very content until two years earlier.

113

L.D. was the youngest child in her family and had a demanding, temperamental older sister who caused much turmoil. L.D. had become a good, helpful child who did chores without being asked and never caused family upsets. She was close to her mother and they confided in each other. At age 17 L.D. left home for further training, and when she returned a few years later she felt she had lost her place to a young cousin who had come to live with the family. After several months L.D. left home again to work, and met and married her husband.

L.D.'s husband's job involved several moves far from her home town and she saw little of her parents. She became very involved in community work and running a small business. People knew her as someone they could always turn to, and she was kept very busy. One neighbor in particular began to call her frequently for help in resolving marital crises. Soon L.D. found herself spending a great deal of time with this woman and began to tell her things she had never revealed to anyone before. L.D. was available whenever her friend had a new marital stress and in return was admired and encouraged to reveal herself.

L.D.'s mother died suddenly and her husband was unable to accompany her to the funeral, so the friend did so instead. L.D. resented her husband's absence while knowing he could not come. She and her friend shared their disappointments in their spouses. L.D. became aware for the first time that she did not wish to be physically near her husband and moved out of the bedroom.

Shortly thereafter L.D. and her friend spent a weekend at a summer cottage. The friend had arranged a candlelight dinner complete with wine and music to greet her arrival. Later that night L.D. "found" herself sexually involved with her friend. Her somatic complaints began almost immediately and she became so debilitated that her doctor put her in the hospital. There she refused visitors and struggled to come to terms with her feelings. She realized that she wanted the friendship of this woman but not sex with her. L.D. began to question how all of this had happened to her.

The case above illustrates the woman's need for caring and intimacy, to be loved and accepted for herself, not just as a good girl. L.D. had never allowed such closeness in her marriage but had derived gratification from helping others. Her new friend was able to penetrate her defenses and to manipulate her needs into a sexual affair. As a result, L.D. was forced into self-examination and recognition of her long use of denial and sublimation.

Conclusion

Sexual behavior after separation or divorce is very complex in its origins. For some, it is often an affirmation of desirability, sexuality, femininity; however, it is also indicative of the state of the development of their capacity for intimacy and trust. Homosexual activity may become a part of postdivorce adjustment, as women are found to provide the understanding, sensitivity, and caring required to restore a wounded ego. For other women, the trauma of separation or of the events of the marriage itself force a confrontation of their own lesbian identity.

In general, women associate sexuality with intimacy and find libido to be closely associated with the degree of warmth and closeness that exists in a relationship. This chapter has focused on that association, and has pointed out sociocultural and individual psychological development aspects that strongly influence it.

References

1. Meyers JK: The clinical spectrum of sexual disorders, in Clinical Management of Sexual Disorders (second edition). Edited by: Meyer JK, Schmidt CW Jr, Wise TN. Baltimore, Williams & Wilkins, 1983
2. Erikson E: Identity: Youth and Crisis. New York, W.W. Norton, 1968
3. Money J: Love Maps. New York, Irvington Publishers, 1986
4. Jacobson GF: The multiple crisis of marital separation and divorce, in Seminars in Psychiatry. Edited by Greenblatt M. New York, Grune and Stratton, 1983

5. Cauhape E: Fresh Starts: Men and Women After Divorce. New York, Basic Books, 1983
6. Solomon BM: In the Company of Educated Women. New Haven, CT, Yale University Press, 1985
7. Greatrex TES: Separation and divorce: crisis and development, in Treatment Intervention in Human Sexuality. Edited by Nadelson CC, Marcotte DB. New York, Plenum Press, 1983
8. Nelson JB: Religious and moral issues in working with homosexual clients. J Homosex 7:163-175, 1982

Chapter 6

The Impact of Parental Divorce on Children and Adolescents

ELISSA P. BENEDEK, M.D.

Chapter 6

The Impact of Parental Divorce on Children and Adolescents

*T*he period of parental separation and divorce has become a focus of study for a variety of mental health professionals who work with children and their families. In 1960, fewer than 10 out of 1,000 marriages ended in divorce. In 1983, there were 1,179,000 divorces granted in the United States (1). The divorce rate has more than doubled from 1960 to 1981 (2). Currently, 22.5 percent of all children in this country are living in single-parent homes (3, 4). These single-parent homes are due to divorce.

Divorce is considered one of the most severe psychological stressors for children, a reputation it well deserves (5). The census statistics above underestimate the actual number of children who have experienced parental divorce, since remarriage is not considered in the totals. It has been estimated that 85 percent of divorced adults remarry (three out of four women and five out of six men) and that 40 percent of adults who divorce experience a second divorce (2, 6). Hetherington projected that 40 to 50 percent of children in the United States born in the 1970s would spend some time living in single-parent families because of divorce (7). Those projections continue in the 1980s. Moreover, the demographic data about the number of divorces do not include the 23 to 30 percent of divorce petitions that are withdrawn where a periodic parental separation occurs.

Despite the increasing prevalence of parental separation and divorce and the increasing professional attention paid to the period of separation, divorce, and postdivorce arrangements for children, including custody arrangements (sole or joint custody) and visitation arrangements, conclusive research is lacking concerning many of the variables surrounding divorce and the aftermath. For example, it is not clear whether parental separation per se or the quality of separation (that is, whether it is rancorous or not) and the tempestuous divorce act as temporary stressors or long-term stressors on children. It is also not clear what the relationship of the chronological or developmental age of a child at the time of separation and divorce is to the future mental health or mental illness of the child. It is not clear what effects parental mental illness, emotional disorder, alcoholism, or other addictions have on the short-term accommodation or long-term development of these children. Some clinicians even suggest that parental divorce may not be a significant stressor but rather may lead to increased maturity, better coping mechanisms, stronger interpersonal skills, and better mental health in children (8, 9). In this chapter, I shall review some of the extant longitudinal studies that touch on the long-term adjustment of children and divorce. Also the newer research is reviewed with regard to such variables as sex, age of child, socioeconomic status, quality of pre- and postdivorce interaction of parents, and mental health outcome subsequent to divorce.

Overview

In 1969, Phoebe Ellsworth and Robert Levy, in the course of the development of the Uniform Marriage and Divorce Act, reviewed at length the available research on divorce families and children in other than two-parent settings to determine what was empirically known about the effects of various custodial awards and arrangements on children's development (10). They were disappointed. They did not find studies comparing children of different ages in different custodial settings after divorce. In fact, they could not locate any studies of children living with natural fathers after divorce or any studies of children living with natural mothers who had not been their primary caretakers before divorce. They did find a wealth of studies about children who lived in institutions and children who lived with their natural mothers who had always been their primary caretakers in single-parent families.

On the average, the studies suggested these children were more "troubled" and "more troubling" than children in two-parent homes. Boys especially were reported to have problems of cognitive development, sex role identifications, and delinquency. In the 17 years since Ellsworth and Levy's study, the amount of research on children of divorce has multiplied. However, we are still far from learning all we need to know, and certainly all that would be clinically relevant to prediction of mental health outcome vis-à-vis custodial and visitation arrangements.

Measurement, whether biased or not, is a particular problem in research on this topic. Much of the research on divorce makes use of unstandardized interviews or paper-and-pencil measures that do not have demonstrated reliability or validity. Furthermore, the content of the measurements has often been restricted. Congruent with the expectations that divorce must create psychological problems for children, researchers have mainly focused on assessing pathological domains of children's functioning. Assessment of weaknesses—aggression, disruptions in sex role development, and intellectual deficits—has been common; almost completely overlooked is assessment of the potential impact of divorce on developing strengths such as increased prosocial behavior, independence, sensitivity to the feelings of others, or the ability to cope well with stress (9, 11).

Two studies have been particularly influential on clinicians and in social policy formation because they have been long-term developmental studies. The authors have been prolific both in their initial report and their follow-up reports and have contributed substantially to the literature in this area. Brief descriptions of both studies follow.

The first, by Hetherington, Cox, and Cox (12) was a follow-up study of 72 nursery-school-age children in 48 families over a two-year period following legal divorce. These authors report that in the first few years following divorce, children in families of divorce in comparison to children in nondivorce families show more antisocial impulsive acting out disorders; more aggression and noncompliance; more dependency, anxiety, and depression; more difficulties in social relationships; and more problems in school compared with children in nondivorce families. They noted that at young ages there is more externalizing behavior, impulsive antisocial behavior, and less withdrawal, depression, and anxiety. They comment that these effects are more severe and enduring for young boys than for young girls.

The second study, by Wallerstein and Kelly (13–17), followed 131 children of all ages from 60 middle-upper class families for a 10-year period after separation and divorce. The Wallerstein and Kelly reports are the most extensive clinical interviews of young children, latency children, and adolescent children over a period of time. Young children are described as being frightened, bewildered, and very sad. They have great difficulty in understanding what is happening to them as their family disrupts. For example, I have repeatedly heard children say that their father has "died" or "has gone on a long vacation" or "has gone to visit Jesus."

Young children have a limited capacity to understand reality and that capacity is generally augmented by a rich active fantasy life. In addition, even in today's society where children are privy to many family secrets, parents are reluctant to provide young children with the real facts about parental separation. In an absence of concrete information, children tend to fill a vacuum with fantasy or confabulation. Thus, a combination of an immature cognitive system, a rich imagination, and an absence of fact results in an active process of denial that causes young children to have confused, distorted, and bizarre pictures of what is really happening in their families at a highly emotional level.

In response to anxiety, very young children also regress. For example, they may return to their security blanket, have lapses in toilet training, and show increased masturbatory activity. Young children also tend to feel guilty and blame themselves for the divorce. It is not unusual for the young child to feel that his or her bad behavior has forced an absent parent to leave. A minor misdeed is magnified disproportionately and is seen as the true cause of the parent leaving. Thus, many children remember with clarity the night before daddy left and can talk in a convincing fashion about what *they* did that was wrong.

Wallerstein and Kelly also comment about the rise in aggression in about half of the young children whom they saw. Aggression may be shown as greater irritability toward brothers, sisters, parents, or school, or may be played out in fantasy with animals who beat each other to death or eat other little animals. McDermott, too, reports on the increase in aggressive hostile acting out by boys who bite, destroy toys, and show disorganized flailing behavior that may even be dangerous to other children (18). Sudden transformation of children from models to monsters around the time of parental divorce may be a reenactment of aggressive violent behavior observed at home, an identification with an aggressor, or an attempt to deal with overwhelming affect (anxiety, depression, or guilt) that cannot yet be translated into words. In a clinical population, this aggression may be seen as diffuse aggressive acting out displayed with puppets, toys, or direct aggression to a therapist.

Mental Health Referrals

There is little doubt that children from divorced families are proportionately overrepresented in the outpatient psychiatric and psychological treatment populations. Several studies of clinics in various geographic regions in the United States have revealed that between two and four times as many children from divorced households are brought for treatment as would be expected from the prevalence of divorce in the general population (18–21). Furthermore, these referrals do not appear to be made simply as a reaction to the immediate crisis precipitated in a family at the time of divorce: According to the findings of one investigation, treatment referrals are made an average of five years following the divorce (21). Thus, the children of divorce appear to be at increased risk for general long-term emotional difficulties, at least as indexed or measured by outpatient clinic referrals.

Probably the best estimate of the increased risk for postdivorce childhood psychological problems comes from the one study that was conducted on a nationally representative sample. Zill, in a stratified probability sample of 1,747 U.S. households, found that 14 percent of the children in divorced homes were described by their parents as needing psychological help in the past year, and 13 percent of the children in the sample had actually seen a psychologist or psychiatrist at some point (22, 23). Comparable figures for children in two-parent families were 6 percent identified as needing help and 5½ percent said to have been in treatment.

However, one must interpret any figures on treatment referral cautiously, because, as noted earlier, both current parental reports of mental health problems and treatment referrals may well have been influenced by the divorced parents' expectations that their children would experience psychological problems as a consequence of the divorce and a prevailing similar bias in professionals. Zill's study, which identified an increased risk for general psychological problems among the children of divorced, remains the best current general estimate. Although these data suggest that divorce may be associated with a doubling or tripling of the rate of perceived psychological problems among children, it is important to keep in mind that the data also indicate that over 85 percent of American children are seen by their parents as coping with divorce sufficiently well so as not to need psychological help. However, 85 percent may be an overly optimistic estimate because of the self-report nature of the study.

Problems of Developmental Stages

Young School-Age Children (Six to Eight Years Old)

Wallerstein and Kelly describe the demonstration of grief and sadness of children who have had a serious loss (15). The children may manifest their grief and sadness by crying and sobbing in overt signs of depression. They may also withdraw and exhibit somatic signs of depression, for example, stomachaches or headaches. In addition, children in early latency continue to believe that they are responsible for the parental divorce and that their behavior led to the family disorganization. These children, too, try to master a devastating event through fantasy, particularly fantasies of reconciliation. Such fantasies may be expressed in play or directly.

Late Latency–Early Adolescent Children

Wallerstein and Kelly describe older children, 9 to 12 years old, as seeming to be able to express more anger in a more direct, conscious, mature way (16). The anger is well organized and object directed, at the father, the mother, both parents, the grandparents, or significant others. In the main, these children were described as being angry at the parent whom they blamed for the divorce. (That parent may not be responsible.) Older, latency-aged children are more likely to align themselves with one or the other of the parents. They may align with the parent of the same sex as a form of identification or with the parent of the opposite sex. The alignment may be their own internal response caused by external measures.

Adolescence

Adolescents are described as feeling less guilty and being more reality oriented at the time of parental separation. Many authors note that the average adolescent tends to recognize that it is not his or her behavior alone that is responsible for the parental friction. Indeed, many adolescents may be the prover-

125

bial straw that broke the camel's back, but adolescents feel much less guilty about their contribution to the parental crisis. They tend to look at parental behavior surrounding divorce in a more objective way. Adolescents seem to be more concerned about the realities, such as who will pay for their clothes, their schooling, and their medical bills. Other realities like who is sleeping with whom and when and where adulterous activities occur tend to become the focus of their conversations with their peers and parents and a source of fantasy. Adolescents are preoccupied with their own future. Foreshadowing of a concern that will follow them into later life is the adolescent concern about relations with the opposite sex. Wallerstein and Kelly note that adolescents worry about the reasons for their parent's inability to have a lasting sexual relationship with a person of the opposite sex and wonder if that inability will be transmitted genetically or environmentally to them. Some adolescents enter into a premature sexual relationship with a person who is very similar in appearance or temperament to the parent they have lost through divorce.

Sex Differences in Social and Emotional Development

A number of researchers have commented on the more obvious early and long-lasting difficulties in boys (13, 24). It is believed that boys are more likely to exhibit aggressive or acting out behavior in response to stress. This may be a biological predisposition as a result of socialization. The difference might also be related to problems of identification and parental control of boys living with the opposite-sex parent (25). Girls, on the other hand, seem to internalize problems and be more protected until early adolescence.

Long-Term Studies

Both Hetherington et al. and Wallerstein have conducted long-term studies of children and divorce (12, 14). Hetherington et

126

al. were able to follow their original group of nursery school children six years after the parental divorce, when the children were an average of 10.1 years old. They note that six years later many rearrangements in family life have occurred. An obvious caveat in studying these children is that the status and mental health of the child are related to the many intervening variables, including changes in economic status, residence, parental occupation, child care arrangements, social relationships, support networks, family relationships, physical and mental health of the child, and family members. Such changes are often related to an adjustment in psychological well-being of children. Hetherington et al. were able to obtain measures of child adjustment from parents, teachers, peers, and the child. All of the measures were selected or constructed to measure internalizing, externalizing, and socially competent behavior. In summary, Hetherington et al. note that their findings are in agreement with findings of earlier studies that divorce has more adverse long-term effects on boys.

They also note that the remarriage of a custodial mother is associated with an increase in behavior problems in girls and some decrease in problems in boys. Although the boys in stepparent families are not as well adjusted as sons in nondivorced families, they are better adjusted in the long run than those who remain in divorced mother-headed households. It seems that divorced mothers and sons who are often involved in mutual patterns of coercion have much to gain from the addition of a responsive, authoritative stepfather who offers support to both the mother and son. Children often benefit from the presence of an involved same-sex stepparent. In contrast, divorced mothers and their daughters often have formed close relationships that the intrusion of a stepfather may disrupt. Stepfathers, too, may view their relationships with stepchildren as a major problem in their marriage. Stepfathers report more problem behaviors in their stepchildren, especially in their stepdaughters, than do the mothers and the children. It may be that the budding sexuality of a preteen has particular disruptive effects in a reconstituted family.

In answer to the question of whether children who have problems in the preschool years and two years postdivorce continue to show the same problems four years later, Hetherington et al. comment, "This seems to depend on the sex of the child, the ensuing family reorganization, and the negative life experiences encountered by the child. There is less continuity in the adjustment of children from divorced families than in nondivorced families because of the greater probability they have of encountering multiple negative life family changes in such things as family relationships, mental and physical health of the family members, child care, geographic mobility, and economic status" (12). They do emphasize that "early aggressive and antisocial behavior is more predictive of later behavioral problems and lack of social competence than is early withdrawal and anxiety predictive of long-term withdrawal or anxiety." Moreover, early externalizing behavior in girls, because it is less frequent and less sex appropriate (or aggressive antisocial), is the best predictor of later socially inept behavior (aggressive antisocial). In contrast, early social competence in girls shows only a modest relationship to later social skills in female adolescents. Much greater stability in social competence over time is found in boys. Preschool boys who are viewed by peers, teachers, and parents as socially unskilled and insensitive are less competent and show more antisocial behavior in later years.

Wallerstein, too, has studied children 10 years subsequent to divorce (14). (Her group is an older group.) She was able to locate and interview members in 87 percent of the original 56 families. As mentioned earlier, Wallerstein was able to study these same children 18 months following the parental separation, again in 5 years, and yet again at 10 years postseparation. At 18 months following the marital separation, psychological decline was noted among all the children and adolescents who at least superficially had seemed to survive the failing marriage. A difference between the sexes emerged early. Young boys below the age of adolescence were significantly more troubled in their performance and behavior at school, playground, and home than were girls. In fact, many of the girls initially seemed to be well on their way to recovery. It should be noted that almost all of the youngsters Wallerstein studied had mothers who were in a custodial process.

At the end of the five-year mark, Wallerstein noted that the most important predictor of a good adjustment in the children was the overall quality of life within the postdivorce family. Neither the age of the child at the time of the marital separation nor the sex of the child was significant in outcome. The quality of parenting within the postdivorce family, the continuity of relationships with the visiting parent, and the extent to which the conflict had subsided all contributed to the well-being in the child. At five years, Wallerstein continued to note the persistence of anger at the parent who initiated the divorce, the intensity of longing for the absent or visiting parent, the persistence of the youngster's wish to reconstitute the predivorce family. She noted the number of children who were markedly psychologically disturbed, particularly showing a severe clinical depression.

At 10 years, Wallerstein returned to evaluate the same population, and the following factors seemed to be important in the 40 young men and women of the original sample. About half of the adolescents were in school (college or graduate school), but half were entirely out of school. The youngsters who had dropped out of school before graduation from high school were all girls. Of the youngsters entirely out of school, three were unemployed and had few marketable skills. The rest were employed in itinerant or relatively unskilled jobs such as waitressing or temporary sales positions. In contrast to comparable youngsters in the same community, only two-thirds were attending or had graduated from college (compared to 85 percent of the youngsters in the upper middle class community studied), and those who were in school received very little help, financial or emotional, from their fathers (the noncustodial parent).

Even more striking, of the 40 young people, 27 (or 68 percent of the group) had engaged in mild to serious illegal activity during their adolescence or young adulthood. Their delinquency ranged from underaged alcohol consumption or recreational drug use to serious illegal activities including assault, burglary, arson, drug dealing, and theft. The type of offense differed between the sexes. Only three of the girls had engaged in serious delinquent activity, which included prostitution, burglary, and physical assault. The young men were more likely to be involved in serious antisocial acts.

Of the 40 young men and women, 6 women and 3 men were already in second marriages. The women married at 17, 18, and 19 years of age. One woman married at 18, divorced at 21, and remarried at 22. One-third of all the women had been pregnant outside of the marriage. One-quarter of those women had elected to have abortions and two women had had two abortions. These findings support Wallerstein and Kelly's (16) concerns about premature sexual behavior and marriage in an attempt to resolve conflicts that were initiated at the time of divorce. These young adults are still demonstrating feelings of sadness and depression. They cried as they recalled their past and their memories of the separation. In these youngsters time did not mute painful feelings and memories.

The young adults also felt that they had sustained an important loss. Two-thirds of them remarked that they had lost the experience of growing up within the protection and emotional nurturance of an intact family. They shared a sense of being deprived or needy. They felt that life for them had been more difficult, more hazardous, less pleasurable than for their peers whose families remained intact. They told the interviewers that the divorce continued to hold a moderately or high central position in their psychological functioning. A common comment was "My life would have been happier if my parents hadn't divorced. Divorce was better for them but not for me. I lost my family; I lost the experience of growing up in a family unit."

Despite the sense of loss, most of these late adolescents/young adults were no longer angry. Those who were were angry at what they considered their parents' immoral behavior during the marriage. Many of these young people embraced a morality that was more traditional than that of their parents. They continued to condemn their parents for what they viewed as irresponsible or immoral conduct in the past. They were strongly against marital infidelity, and they stressed the importance of choosing correctly the first time around. To the problem of correct choice, many of them envisioned a solution of living with a lover for several years prior to a marriage, knowing that person very well, then waiting a while to be absolutely sure of a lasting relationship before children were conceived.

Wallerstein, too, notes the importance of sibling relationships. Although these young men and women had lost a parent, many of them became especially close to their brothers and sisters and used their brothers and sisters as a powerful support system who could buffer the family ordeal and provide nourishment to them in a time of stress.

The more troublesome effect of divorce on young boys, and later-latency and adolescent girls, is reported by other observers. Kalter describes young women from divorced families as carrying "a delayed time bomb," a time bomb which leads to many symptomatic responses, including precocious sexual activity, substance abuse, and running away from home (19, 20). These findings are also reported in a "normal" population, not the population that presents itself in the clinical setting.

Conclusion

What then do we know, on the basis of research and clinical experience, about children's and adolescents' reaction to divorce, and how can we be of help to them? First, there are long-term and lasting effects in the nonclinic population of divorced children. Second, brief supportive psychotherapy (13) does not help to prevent lasting effects. Third, the long-term effects seem to be most severe in girls. And fourth, visitation and regular visitation patterns seem to be prophylactic in regard to preventing long-term problems. The implication for social policy and mental health treatment for children seems obvious: A social policy is needed that encourages contact with a noncustodial parent because such contact is critical to the future of the child.

References

1. National Center for Health Statistics: Births, Marriages, Divorces and Deaths for 1983. Monthly Vital Statistics Report, March 26, 1984 (PHS 84-1220)
2. Cherlin AJ: Marriage, Divorce, Remarriage. Cambridge, MA, Harvard University Press, 1981
3. U.S. Bureau of Census: Current Population Reports, Series P-20, No. 371: Household and Family Characteristics: March 1981. Washington, DC, U.S. Government Printing Office, 1982
4. U.S. Bureau of the Census: Current Population Report Series P-20, No. 372: Marital Status and Living Arrangements: March 1981. Washington, DC, U.S. Government Printing Office, 1982
5. American Psychiatric Association: Diagnostic and Statistical Manual of Mental Disorders (Third Edition-Revised). Washington, DC, American Psychiatric Association, 1987
6. Moss SZ, Moss MS: Surrogate mother–child relationships. Am J Orthopsychiatry, 45:382-390, 1975
7. Hetherington EM: Divorce: a child's perspective. Am Psychol 34:851-858, 1979
8. Bane MJ: Here to Stay: American Families in the 20th Century. New York, Basic Books, 1976
9. Hetherington EM: Divorce, children and social policy, in Child Development Research and Social Policy. Edited by Stevenson HW, Siegel AE. Chicago, University of Chicago Press, 1984
10. Ellsworth P, Levy R: Legislative reform of child custody adjudication: an effort to rely on social science data in formulating legal policies. Law and Society Review 4:167-169, 1969

11. Emery RE: Interparental conflict and children of discord and divorce. Psychol Bull 92:310-330, 1982

12. Hetherington EM, Cox R: Effects of divorce on parents and children in nontraditional families: parenting and child development, in Nontraditional Families. Edited by Lamb M. Hillsdale, NJ, Erlbaum, 1982

13. Wallerstein JS, Kelly JB: Surviving the Breakup: How Children Actually Cope with Divorce. New York, Basic Books, 1980

14. Wallerstein JS: Children of divorce: preliminary report of a ten year follow-up of older children and adolescents. J Am Acad Child Psychiatry 245:545-553, 1985

15. Wallerstein JS, Kelly JB: The effects of parental divorce: experiences of the pre-school child. J Am Acad Child Psychiatry 14:600-616, 1975

16. Wallerstein JS, Kelly JB: The effects of parental divorce: experiences in the child in later latency. Am J Orthopsychiatry 46:256-269, 1976

17. Wallerstein JS, Kelly JB: The effects of parental divorce: the adolescent experience, in Children at Psychiatric Risk (Vol. 3). Edited by Anthony EJ, Koupernick C. New York, Wiley, 1974

18. McDermott JF: Divorce and its psychiatric sequellae in children. Arch Gen Psychiatry 23:421-427, 1970

19. Kalter N: Children of divorce in an outpatient psychiatric population. Am J Orthopsychiatry 47:40-51, 1977

20. Kalter N, Rembar J: The significance of a child's age at the time of parental divorce. Am J Orthopsychiatry 51:85-100, 1981

21. Tuckman J, Regan RA: Intactness of the home and behavioral problems in children. J Child Psychol Psychiatry 7:225-233, 1966

22. Zill N: Divorce, marital happiness and the mental health of children: findings from the F.C.D. national survey of children. Paper presented at the National Institute of Mental Health Workshop on Divorce and Children, Bethesda, MD. February, 1978

133

23. Zill N: Happy, Healthy and Insecure. New York, Doubleday, 1983
24. Cadoret RJ, Cain C: Sex differences in predictors of antisocial behavior in adoptees. Arch Gen Psychiatry 37:1171-1175, 1980
25. Santrock J, Warshak R: Father custody and social adjustment in boys and girls. Journal of Social Issues 35:112-115, 1979

*From the Trees
to the Forest:
What Developmental
Approaches to Divorce
Offer the Matrimonial
Lawyer*

R. JAMES WILLIAMS, L.L.B., M.S.W., B.Sc.

Chapter 7

From the Trees to the Forest: What Developmental Approaches to Divorce Offer the Matrimonial Lawyer

Divorce, the legal termination of a marriage, has become easier to obtain in most North American jurisdictions in recent years, with a steady movement toward "no fault" divorce. At the same time, the law has become increasingly complex in its treatment of issues that are corollary to divorce—custody, maintenance payments, and division of property.

In the area of custody there are developments such as joint custody, shared parenting, mediation, representation of children, and questions and reevaluation regarding issues such as mobility of custodial parents, the extent of parental rights, religion, race, differences in parenting styles, the relationship between maintenance and access, the usefulness of the tender years doctrine, the concepts of bonding and status quo, the role of grandparents and extended family, the role of expert witnesses, and the extent of children's rights.

With respect to maintenance, we have seen a change in the way the family *and roles within the family* are perceived.

There are obligations on each spouse to attempt to become self-sufficient. Marriage is not necessarily seen as a lifelong commitment, nor is maintenance. Some individuals, in my experience most often middle-aged or older women, are left after a divorce with expectations of self-sufficiency that are totally foreign to their own values and expectations, which were that marriage and/or the right to support were lifelong things. These people are trapped by a value system that was totally legitimate in their formative years and a society that has since changed the rules.

What is fair maintenance? What should be done with or for the spouse who is marginally employed? For the spouse who is a middle or upper income earner? Should there be a "topping up" of maintenance based on life-style? How long should maintenance last? Should education or upgrading of the spouse be paid for by maintenance? Who should evaluate whether it is a legitimate or prudent course of study? How long should maintenance last? Should maintenance be paid rather than have an unmotivated, emotionally paralyzed or disabled spouse go on welfare? What is the relationship between first and second families—how can the law balance or give priority to one or the other? What consideration should be given to the impact of a new relationship (for either spouse) and the income of that new person in assessing maintenance? What role, if any, does conduct during or after the marriage have in maintenance?

What property is matrimonial and subject to division? Gifts, business interests, inheritances, professional degrees or practices, property acquired before or after the marriage, pensions, insurance proceeds, debts, loans (especially with extended family), and numerous other areas present special problems. How is the division to be made? On what considerations? What of unmarried "spouses"? Of what relevance are conduct? earning capacity? arrangements with respect to children or elderly family members?

The questions that the matrimonial lawyer must deal with have become increasingly complex. The development of no-fault divorce and deemphasis of conduct with respect to corollary issues has meant that institutionally the law and the lawyer are less focused on the marital breakup itself. Consequently, the lawyer, in advising a client, may become less inclined to explore and attempt to understand the client's personal "process" as it relates to the marriage and the marital relationship.

The divorce lawyer is generally seen by the client as an expert. The problems and considerations attendant to the resolution of custody, maintenance, and property issues arising from the dissolution of a marriage transcend categorization as "legal" problems. According to Hancock (1), "Clients endow their attorneys with power relating to the social, psychological and emotional dimensions of their lives, quite apart from the counselor's conception of the legal role and its limits" (p. 235). Questions and issues such as "What is reasonable access?", "What should I tell the kids?", "Do I have to give half the family photos?", "Should I get out of the car when I drop the kids off?", "Do I have to apply for jobs clerking?", "Can I date? Can I be sexually active?", "Should I stop seeing my psychiatrist?", and "Should I start seeing a psychiatrist?" make this obvious.

The lawyer faced with such questions must attempt to answer them in large part based on information obtained from one side of a two- or multisided (where there are children) problem.

At the same time, the traditional training and approach of lawyers is to analyze situations and advise clients on a case-by-case, problem-by-problem basis. This to a great extent is the proper role for the lawyer. The result, however, is that the lawyer, often anxious not to be a counselor, may not see his client as a person undergoing an emotional and social process. However, an awareness of this will assist the lawyer in assessing the client and providing him or her with informed, effective advice with respect to both short- and long-term consequences of decisions of courses of action.

Psychosocial Aspects of Divorce

Examining divorce in a process-oriented or developmental fashion can only assist the lawyer in broadening his or her knowledge, awareness, and, in the end, the effectiveness of his or her advice. The divorce client is seeking advice about both the legal and nonlegal consequences of the divorce. There is a considerable amount of literature and commentary on divorce and the divorce process from the developmental perspective. Inherent in these approaches is a recognition that the legal divorce is a *symbolic disengagement* of a commitment to a joint relationship. It is not necessarily a disengagement from a relationship with an ex-spouse, the spouse's family, friends, or the emotions, memories, and attachments that developed within the marriage. These "nonlegal" analyses of divorce differ in focus. Some look at "areas of impact," that is, areas of one's life that are affected; some examine divorce in terms of a personality process, development, or reaction; and some look at social implications.

Social science and developmental analysis of divorce cannot provide the lawyer with a template for divorce. Individuals are too different to allow this. The development of models, theories, or phases should be seen not as an attempt to categorize, but rather as a mechanism to increase understanding and stimulate reflection and thought about the lawyer's role. Inevitably, broadened knowledge or appreciation of divorce will assist the lawyer in recognizing a client's needs and limitations. The issues that the lawyer deals with cut across multiple disciplines, and it is not unrealistic to expect the lawyer to have some knowledge of the approach of these various disciplines to divorce.

A brief review of Bohannan's six stations of divorce, the grief model, and Saunders's discussion of social consequences of divorce will serve to illustrate some of this nonlegal literature and its potential benefits to the lawyer in providing an awareness of the broader view.

Bohannan's Model

I would view Bohannan's "six stations of divorce" (2) as an "area of impact" analysis. His "stations" are not stages but areas of experience that occur within most divorces though differing in order or intensity. These stages are described in the following sections.

The Emotional Divorce

Discontent, dissatisfaction, the erosion of trust, development of ambivalence, and withholding of emotion become visible in the relationship. The relationship may be salvageable through counseling or reconciliation if neither party has "let go" of the relationship. The divorce lawyer is in a position to reinforce, and may do so positively or negatively (in terms of the relationship). The lawyer's response to described difficulties will vary between responses such as "We'll get that s.o.b." and "It sounds like you and your spouse are not communicating," and he or she will influence the client's attitude to reconciliation, mediation, and/or divorce itself.

The Legal Divorce

This station refers to the legal process itself and, inherently, the lawyer–client relationship. The lawyer should be aware of any personal biases that he or she may have and should communicate these to the client, for example, a bias for or against mediation or joint custody. The lawyer's reputation and personality will no doubt contribute to the nature of his or her clientele—the "fighter," "negotiator," "husband's," "wife's," "custody," "do anything," and "reasonable" reputations are examples. The lawyer should have some ideas as to what preconceptions the client has had in choosing him or her and what this might mean in terms of the client's expectations for the legal process. The lawyer will create expectations too, and although the lawyer who makes rash or exaggerated promises about financial or custodial results may initially keep a client, he or she also sets limits and boundaries for subsequent negotiations.

There is little that will more effectively ensure bitterness and litigation than the improvident, unrealistic raising of expectations by a lawyer. Subsequent negotiations, if based on realistic *judicial* guidelines, will be met with "But you said . . ." and will undermine trust between lawyer and client. The alternative is that having created unrealistic expectations, the lawyer lets the client go into litigation with unrealistic demands. One way of creating trust in the client is for the lawyer to acknowledge that he or she does not have all of the answers, is not always right, and is not averse to clients seeking second opinions. This also allows the lawyer to deal with the client who seems firm in a course of action that is, in the view of the lawyer, detrimental to the client.

The lawyer should recognize that there are times when legal advice or actions will serve to aggravate emotions, for example, advising a spouse seeking custody not to leave the home or writing inflammatory or accusatory letters. The lawyer should also be aware of any emotions he or she may have regarding the other lawyer involved in the divorce: If there is dislike, respect, or any other regard between counsel, it will influence the process accordingly.

The Economic Divorce

The economic divorce relates to financial issues: spousal and child support and the property settlements. Expectations are, as already discussed, easily created whether by the lawyer or that familiar but never seen "friend that got everything" (or paid nothing). Each situation and circumstance is different. A husband's counsel can take a step toward instilling trust in a distrustful wife or wife's counsel with full, frank, immediate disclosure, provision of postdated maintenance checks (avoiding the aggravation of waiting for the check or temptation to jerk an ex-spouse's chain by sending it late). Often seemingly minor pieces of property acquire great importance by reason of sentimentality or symbolism.

The painting that becomes the symbol of "winning" should be recognized as such by counsel and, if possible, be used to more effectively allow the client to negotiate. Counsel may explain that he and his spouse seem to be viewing the painting as "winning," that if we let her "win" we may be able to achieve something more substantial, that it is good to let her feel she "won" or was successful because then there is less likelihood of a change of mind or application to court to vary an agreement or order.

There are a number of issues relating to "self-sufficiency" and maintenance that have been referred to at the beginning of this chapter, and the lawyer should strive to understand and be explicit about the expectations that are created for individual clients or their spouses.

The Co-Parental Divorce

This station relates to custody and access issues. They may become intertwined with economic issues ("I need the house and furniture and support for the children"). The children maintain, or should maintain, relationships with each parent. Joint custody and shared custody are concepts that have grown out of recognition of this. Where there are children it is obvious that the divorced couple must maintain a relationship after the divorce. They are tied together by the children and the needs of the children. The manipulation and/or exploitation of children is a danger, and perhaps to a degree a reality, inherent in all custody litigation. Ideally the lawyer will discourage it. Whether it is called joint custody, shared parenting, or access, contact and caregiving by the other parent, apart from benefiting the child, can provide a "break," some privacy, and some freedom for the person who finds himself or herself, as a result of divorce, parenting on his or her own. The maintenance of a meaningful relationship with the noncustodial spouse makes the regular provision of maintenance payments more likely.

Children's reactions to and experience of divorce, may be seen in the following stages (3):

1. Troubled marriage
2. Separation
3. Transition and legal steps
4. Divorce and aftermath

The impact of these can be differentiated with reference to the age of the child (6). The lawyer will frequently be left in the position of being asked, "What should I tell the children?" The responsible lawyer will have some familiarity with the literature referred to, appreciate the individual children, be concerned about the long- as well as the short-term relationships within the fractured family, and attempt to avoid aggravating an already stressful situation for the child. The involvement of social work or psychological or psychiatric advice will at times be warranted.

The law has struggled with "the wishes or preferences" of children and how to receive or weigh them. The lawyer should be cognizant of the background contributing to such wishes. The seven-year-old who has been provided with a television, video game, and telephone for his new room with parent A will have "wishes" that should be seen in context. That context will normally include the child's age, stage, and ability to understand temporally and emotionally what is happening. This is applicable to any of the child's behavior.

Allegations of inadequate or improper parenting by the other spouse inevitably have an impact upon the children. There is disturbing growth in the frequency of allegations of sexual abuse of children in marital disputes. Certainly these are not all well founded, and the effect of even the assessment process on the child must be a cause of concern. The effect of such allegations on the parental relationship is obvious. No matter who is the "winner" of the custody dispute, the parents will, except in extraordinary circumstances, have to deal with each other. The potential impact of allegations of any sort, as they relate to parenting, are so great that they should be put forward only upon reflection and preferably where there is independent evidence to substantiate them.

The Community Divorce

The social impact of divorce—the loss of friendship and need to reorganize socially—falls under the Community Divorce station. This may include new or first-time employment or retraining. The client who is looking for a lawyer who will be a "friend" or is becoming emotionally dependent will in most instances result in the lawyer's making, or attempting to make, a referral to a mental health professional.

The Psychic Divorce

The psychic divorce is seen as the successful resolution of the divorce process, the establishment of autonomy from the marriage. The lawyer, through his or her advice and role in the legal divorce, has impact on the client's expectations and postdivorce adjustment.

Grief Model

A variety of authors have related the Kubler-Ross five phases of grief resolution (denial, anger, bargaining, depression, and acceptance) (6) to individual adjustment to divorce (7). Family law lawyers are familiar with clients who at one time or another have displayed modes of

1. Denial—"We'll reconcile, we'll get back together, he still loves me, he'll look after me."
2. Anger—"I don't care what it costs."

3. Bargaining—"I'll change."
4. Depression—"Give her what she wants."
5. Acceptance.

Crosby et al. (7) point out that these feelings and the attendant behavior differ in each individual. They note in particular that there is often, in divorce, "an active and a passive agent" and that the passive agent will be slower to deal with the divorce emotionally. They point out, significantly, that unlike grief resolution, the divorce process involves a significant amount of decision making and individual responsibility. This has significant implications for the family lawyer.

The client whose emotional state intrudes on his or her decision-making ability creates difficulties for the lawyer who is attempting to present alternative courses of action and receive instructions. The client is making decisions that he or she will live with forever. The lawyer will need to recognize when a client's emotions effect or incapacitate his or her ability to give proper instructions. Delay, confrontation, imploring, second opinions, repetition, referral to mental health professionals, and withdrawal as counsel are all used by the lawyer. A sensitivity to the client's divorce process may allow the lawyer to work with the client through a period of emotional exaggeration. It will also allow the lawyer to advise the client, not only in the here and now, but with respect to the future legal and nonlegal consequences of particular courses of action, both in terms of the client and the client's spouse.

Saunders Model

Another approach or analysis of divorce is Saunders's model of the social consequences of divorce (8). Using research on interpersonal consequences (in terms of relationships with family of origin, former spouse, family of former spouse, and friends) as well as activity consequences (work, organizations, hobbies), the Saunders model discloses where a client's support, emotional and/or financial, is likely to come from, what areas of a client's life are changed or are likely to change, and what postdivorce adjustment will be like socially. A client with no social outlets or supports will experience difficulties.

Conclusion

The lawyer, like any professional dealing with a human problem, is dealing with a problem that is multidimensional. The ability to be open to, to assimilate, and to use bodies of knowledge from other disciplines dealing with the same "problem" can only broaden the lawyer's expertise. There is no right or wrong way to advise. It is as individual a process as the client's divorce process. Awareness of developmental approaches to divorce increases the knowledge base of the lawyer, enabling him or her to go beyond the trees to the forest.

References

1. Hancock E: The power of the attorney in divorce. Journal of Family Law 19:235, 1980–1981
2. Bohannan P: The six stations of divorce, in Divorce and After. Edited by Bohannan P. New York, Doubleday, 1980
3. Brenner A: Helping Children Cope with Stress. Lexington, Mass., D.C. Heath, 1984
4. Neal JJ: Children's understanding of their parents' divorce, in Children and Divorce. Edited by Kurdek LA. San Francisco, Jossey-Bass, 1983
5. Wallerstein JS, Kelly JB: Surviving the Break-Up: How Parents and Children Cope with Divorce. New York, Basic Books, 1980
6. Kubler-Ross E: On Death and Dying. New York, MacMillan, 1969
7. Crosby F, Gage A, Raymond MC: The grief process in divorce. Journal of Divorce 7:3, 1983
8. Saunders E: The social consequences of divorce. Journal of Divorce 6:1, 1983

Chapter 8

Divorce as Development: The Process of Psychotherapy

JUDITH H. GOLD, M.D., F.R.C.P.(C)

Chapter 8

Divorce as Development: The Process of Psychotherapy

*T*he previous chapters have explored the causes and effects of divorce for individuals as adults, as children, and as young adults, as well as the particular effects upon men and upon women. We have thus examined divorce through stages of life and socialization. In this chapter, divorce is discussed as a catalyst for interpersonal psychological maturation, aided by the process of therapeutic intervention. The destruction of the marital dyad can result in creative individual growth through the use of insights gained from an examination of the marriage and of the events and emotions around the divorce.

For most, divorce is extremely painful. One scale measuring the severity of 43 life events has rated divorce second only to the death of a spouse (1). Another, based on stressful life events for psychiatric patients, placed divorce and separation 10th and 11th on a scale of 61 events (2). Yet, while bereavement due to death has received much attention in the psychiatric literature, bereavement due to divorce has not. As discussed in the previous chapters, from 40 to 50 percent of marriages culminate in divorce, that is, end in pain and in various kinds of suffering. Thus divorce is a life event. It is more than a crisis, more than an acute situational reaction, but is an upheaval in lives that affects the core of self-esteem and the functioning of an individual.

The affected person often then comes to a therapist for help in dealing with the trauma of the loss of the marriage. In this chapter I shall outline how the stages of reaction to a divorce can become part of a psychodynamically oriented psychotherapy rather than merely crisis intervention.

The Psychological Stages of Divorce

Initial

In North America the family is still thought of in its traditional form of two parents living together with their children. Advertisements reflect this supposition through the use of images of such families, but statistics show that this is more and more an erroneous view of family life today (3, 4). Nevertheless, the young grow up with this expectation of marriage as long lasting and mutually satisfactory. Thus the dissolution of the union has repercussions within a person's sense of identity and self-actualization in our society.

For many, marriage is "forever" and its ending is seen as a personal failure, an inability to sustain a relationship that is evident to all and thus humiliating. Feelings of rejection add to this self-denigration, and the person loses the comfortable boundaries of his or her prior self-image. Some have described the loss of attachment as similar to that of abandonment and related this to Bowlby's description of the bonding between mother and child (5). Certainly, most react with a sense of helplessness associated with an intense feeling of loss. They react much like a child who feels left and forgotten with initial angry crying followed by withdrawal and denial. Much of this behavior is, of course, determined by previous life experiences around the sense of rejection (6). This regression is qualitatively different from that of mourning after the death of a spouse. One woman stated, "It would be easier if he was dead, but he is alive and rejecting me."

In most situations, one partner asks the other for a divorce or decides to leave. The initial reaction to this may be disbelief or shock even if there had been prior indications that all was not well. Occasionally, one or both feel relief, a sense of freedom at being able to do what they please and be alone: "Finally I can come home and there is no one there waiting to argue with me"; "I can keep the place just as I like it"; "I am free to come and go as I please"; and "The baby doesn't have colic anymore" are common statements.

However, the majority of separated persons, including those who voiced the comments above, find this initial tranquillity to be short lived. After a few days to a few weeks the tranquillity is superseded by intense loneliness alternating with uncontrollable crying and/or potentially violent, self-disturbing rages. These emotions are overwhelming and often devastating to the individual, who feels out of control and helpless. The individual may contemplate or attempt suicide in a feeling of hopelessness.

As Hunt wrote, "Of all the negative feelings of the newly separated, none is more common and more important than loneliness; only a minority fail to suffer from it, and even those who most keenly desired the end of the marriage often find the initial loneliness excruciating" (5, p. 125).

During this stage of reaction to the separation, the person may have trouble sleeping and complain of poor concentration and inattention at work. Decision making may be very difficult. Weekends are particularly unpleasant, especially if the child or children are with the other parent and days must be spent alone. Friends and relatives can be strong support systems at this stage, but the person may be reluctant to unburden him- or herself on them. Frequent dreams or obsessive thoughts about the departed spouse may trouble the person during this period.

The events of the marriage are replayed in thought over and over again as the individual searches for "where it went wrong" and "what I should have done differently." These individuals blame themselves for the marriage breakdown and call themselves "a failure." At this point they cannot imagine ever being interested in another again.

This intense reaction can last up to three or four months in some. The length is determined by a number of factors, each of which will be discussed separately.

Prior Socialization

In other chapters of this monograph traditional views of marriage and gender roles have been discussed. Many people marry believing fully that it will be forever. Following the marriage ceremony, the man and woman must learn how to live together. The complexity and need for cooperation, compromises, and consideration for the other are rarely appreciated by the newly wed.

Erikson wrote that young adulthood begins with the ability to tolerate intimacy without fear of loss of self (7). However, more recently it has been noted that this ability develops differently in men than in women (8). Many young men take years to develop a self-concept firm enough to allow true intimacy. They marry feeling they want to share their life with this other person but find that difficult to do once curtailment of, or at least limits on, their own wishes or activities are made necessary by daily responsibilities. Thus many young men still expect to continue all of their former activities with "the guys" while the wife is to wait at home. Or a couple may have many mutual activities that become impossible to share so continually once a child is born. The demands of financial planning, child care, time constraints, and shared attention can become intolerable. The man is attuned to his own needs and cannot make the adaptations necessary, even when children are not part of the marriage.

In contrast, many young women feel a strong need for intimacy well before they develop a strong ego identity. They want to share with and be interdependent. Their identity formation is strongly linked to being married. They expect to be totally involved in the life of their spouse. Such differing needs in a relationship obviously lead to many clashes and potential disasters.

Despite these psychological aspects, many people believe they are indeed married for better or for worse and come from families with the same expectations. Complaints of marital unhappiness may be met with comments from parents such as "You made your bed, now lie in it"; "You can't divorce until the children are grown and on their own"; and "What did you do wrong?" In these circumstances, the newly separated person is unable to obtain emotional support from the family at a time when he or she needs love and reassurance the most. Guilt and self-blame predominate in this individual's initial reaction to the impending divorce.

Psychological Products of the Marriage

The end of a marriage almost always engenders a loss of self-esteem in the initial reactive process. Rejection is a devastating event whether the spouse has left for another person or because the relationship was intolerable to one or both.

When the marriage has been marked by belittlement of the wife, she may have little remaining self-esteem anyway. This is particularly likely when the process was a long assault upon her every thought, action, and reaction, so that she was constantly put down and devalued. This woman may feel totally inadequate and unable to recognize any asset with which to cope. Belittlement of the sort described in Chapter 2 also is demoralizing, but women in this case should have strengths at their outside work upon which to draw while attempting to deal with feelings of abandonment.

Another dimension comes from chronic lack of affection and attention from the spouse who has now departed. The person feels worthless and may find him- or herself unlovable and deserving of this abandonment. Expression of feelings and a display of affect may be found to be difficult after years of neglect and being ignored.

Finally, the process of the marital breakdown may have resulted in a depressive illness. Chapters 3 and 4 contain examples of such cases.

Dependency Needs

Difficulty in absorbing and adjusting to the end of the marriage is related also to the degree of attachment one feels toward the other, as well as toward the institution of marriage, as just discussed above. This attachment may also be rooted differently for men and for women.

A man may view the marriage as a part of, and reflecting, his occupational status and financial achievements to the world. He may see his wife as an integral part of this picture rather than ever having related to her as an individual. Losing her wrecks the vision; it may also make him dramatically aware of her true, but repressed, importance to him psychologically. Further, the loss of his marriage may alter not only where, how, and with whom he lives but is potentially disastrous economically. He may rage that his wife will try to "clean me out, take all I have" and so justify his anger at her. His self-image is damaged in terms of how he thinks he is perceived by others. In addition, he may be astonished and dismayed by his previously unrecognized dependency on his spouse and the degree to which his self-esteem was based on her approval, her existence as his wife, or his need for others to see *her* as *his* wife.

A woman may also have her identity reflected through the marriage, not through using it as a showcase for displaying her own financial achievement, but for displaying her personal emotional, nurturing, and domestic skills. Her self-esteem is built on the involvement she has in her husband's daily and global endeavors and interactions, as well as those of the children, and it will crumble when these are no longer present. If she worked outside of the home, it was usually only for the wages; the important gratification came from her role at home within the marriage. This woman will find a divorce shattering.

Here, too, we must consider the acceptance of a traditional wifely role as a mask over fear of independence and self-sufficiency. She may have been taught, or have learned, that she must be taken care of, that that was a woman's place, or that she was incompetent to take care of herself. She clings to the marriage as to a life-raft and panics when it is removed from her. "The degree of panic during separation speaks to the degree of dependency between partners. The degree of pain speaks to the depth of attachment" (9, p. 330).

In some relationships, one partner, usually the wife, has never dealt with the financial side of living. She may not know what bills arrive each month. She may have never written a check or have had access to family bank accounts. In some cases, she does not know her husband's income or how it is spent or saved. She may not know how to budget money or have any idea of expenses in running their home.

Sometimes one spouse is totally responsible for the physical maintenance of the home or the car. The other may have no idea how to take care of such things and feel helpless to do so. He or she may rage, also, that the spouse allowed this to be so and then left.

Dependency, therefore, has both intrapsychic and practical aspects.

Financial Concerns

The newly separated spouse usually has very real concerns about money. This is complicated when the person is feeling confused, helpless, indecisive, and guilty. The individual may wish to take nothing from the marriage, in a desire to avoid any more arguments, in the belief that the spouse will be fair, or in the belief that he or she does not deserve anything. They may truly believe that the spouse will continue to provide, as always, for them and the children.

A woman may need to find paid employment, using skills from years before or whatever she can find. She struggles to obtain credit, perhaps her own charge cards. She has to pay the household bills and often a mortgage. Suddenly she has all of the responsibility and little of the money. (In Chapters 3 and 4 disputes over money and possessions are detailed.) She may find it very difficult to fight for what she requires while still reacting to the separation itself. Anger may make each spouse unreasonable, as each one fights hurt with anger. Often the departed spouse reacts with anger and uses money as a weapon to wound the other in order to hide guilt and so projects the responsibility for the divorce purely upon the spouse. Children then become involved, since their needs may be neglected as a consequence of the battle. Many men refuse to pay child support because "I don't want to give *her* a cent."

Child Custody Concerns

Either partner may use custody of the child or children as part of the battle to redress wounded self-esteem and to counteract the feelings of rejection and worthlessness. Sometimes custody is disputed not out of love for the child but merely to wound and worry the spouse (see Chapter 3).

These realistic concerns about children and money complicate the critical stage of divorce immensely. The spouse may be furious that the other could neglect their children, while coming slowly to terms with their own separation. Or battles may be fought over visitation rights and other child care decisions, as a vehicle for expressing the rage and distress between them. The custodial parent worries about the effects all of this will have on the child. She may feel badly about and be humiliated by her display of helplessness before her children. She will note that the children seem to be worried about her, that they are doing poorly in school, or that they are disobedient or unusually helpful. (Chapter 6 describes the effect of divorce on children of different ages.) The parent, however, wonders how to provide proper child care and maintain a job and a home alone. She may give up custody early in the divorce process because she feels unworthy and useless, or the demands of child care may aggravate her feelings of denigration and inability to cope.

The Legal Process

Early in the separation, each spouse usually obtains legal advice. In some couples, one spouse cannot afford to do so while the other one can. They may use the same lawyer, believing they can agree on everything. The woman who has lost trust in men due to her interactions with her husband may find it difficult to trust a male lawyer; the dependent, fearful woman may follow legal advice blindly or reject it, fearing it will anger her spouse. The angry husband may instruct his lawyer to be rigid, to delay and harrass, to agree to no financial settlement, and so on. Early on, many are not really able to properly inform their lawyers or to direct them to obtain what they want. The demand for decisions may be unbearable.

Thus, at a very vulnerable time divorcing individuals are faced with many demands, problems, and life-style changes that would be difficult at any time but now just add more burden to their fragile ego functioning.

The Middle Stage

A number of stages of divorce have been described in the literature. Bohannan's six-station divorce process is often referred to, as is Kessler's seven-stage model (10). I prefer to recognize three distinct phases. In the middle period divorcing persons slowly learn to view themselves as separate from the spouse, to detach themselves (11).

In the beginning, they lean heavily on friends and family. Gradually this becomes more difficult, since friends continue to see the other spouse as well or carry tales between the former partners or show less interest. The person feels like an extra at parties and dinners or retreats from yet another introduction to an "available" potential partner. Some fear that friends will tire of them unless they pretend to be cheerful and problem free.

During this stage, all six of the factors described in the previous section continue to weave in and out of daily life, sometimes precipitating crisis after crisis. Difficulties over visitation of the children, especially over predictability of such visits, are usual, as are disputes over property division. Many calls are made to the lawyer, who often appears to be acting with maddening slowness and little explanation. The husband and wife may meet or speak to try to resolve some of these issues themselves and inevitably quarrel bitterly. Occasionally a meeting is pleasant, reviving old memories of warmth and love, and they spend the night or weekend together. This, too, ends in the renewal of fighting, and the episode escalates ambivalence and anger about the divorce.

As discussed in Chapter 5, one or both may become rapidly involved with another or several other people, finding the encounters bolstering to their self-esteem. Some become intensely intimate with another person while still resolving their feelings about the spouse. These relationships are often revealed later to be repetitions of the failed marriage in somewhat altered form. However, the emotional support assists in the battling with the spouse.

Loneliness continues, otherwise, and the person is conscious that something is missing within. One woman stated, "It is like I need a body next to me in bed, any body, just so I am not alone." It is difficult to have no one to share decisions, or problems and joys, or household chores and child care. The parent is constantly responsible for the child or children and feels she never has a day to herself. She may rage that the father is free to do as he pleases, while she must babysit whether she wants to or not. She may have to intercede for young children who wish to communicate with an absent father, further inflaming her resentment.

Financial problems can continue and often worsen. As discussed in Chapter 4, few wives actually receive maintenance for themselves or for the children. Yet there may be requests or demands from paternal relatives to see the children, often while rejecting the wife. She, meanwhile, has to manage a job as well as her work at home. Sometimes she finds a friend in a similar situation to share with, or a student or young relative who will live with her in exchange for helping out with the children. Otherwise, overtime work or a sick child becomes problematic because there is no one else to be with the children or to pick them up from school or daycare.

With all of this going on she is still struggling to regain and establish an identity as an individual. She is now a single person, not someone's wife, and our society has little room for this role beyond adolescence. She must learn to deal with her own sexual needs, as well as with the approaches from others. In short, she is learning to depend on herself and in the process becomes more aware of her inner strengths.

The anger experienced during this stage is sometimes sustained, and at other times becomes sporadic. The person may be shocked to discover how much rage she can feel. She is equally horrified and crushed over and over again by the ongoing behavior of the former spouse toward her. She keeps hoping that he will treat her with consideration and friendship without any evidence of that possibility. These feelings are not limited just to the woman. The person then relives the marital episodes yet again, and the tendency to self-blame and examination continues. Many often develop a variety of physical complaints and visit their family physician for evaluation and treatment.

It is thus obvious that the divorce process resembles that of mourning, with the succession of shock, denial, rage, blame, and finally acceptance and resolution. By the end of this middle stage, which may take several years, the person has come to an acceptance of the divorce and to a new self-knowledge. The legal process, including that of custody and financial concerns, can prolong and intensify the duration of this transition.

Resolution

The stage of resolution is best discussed as part of the process of psychotherapy with the divorcing person.

Psychotherapy

It is well known that women seek help for emotional distress more easily and more frequently than do men. Similarly, when a marriage appears to be breaking down, women turn to professionals for assistance, while their husbands often refuse to attend marital therapy or mediation sessions. The wife may appear, requesting help, at any time in the journey toward the final ending of the marriage.

The initial presenting symptoms may be of anxiety or depression, which may or may not be acknowledged as related to problems in the marriage or from the divorce. In others, the complaint is overwhelming panic attacks or episodes of rage. The connection of these to the marriage may also be unconscious or denied. The stated goal of therapy in these cases is to be relieved of the incapacitating symptoms. Some do request psychotherapy because they wish to be able to deal well with the divorce process or to learn not to repeat past relationships.

Superficially, the required treatment appears to just be psychotherapy for an adjustment disorder, with psychopharmacological intervention as necessary. The therapist must be knowledgeable about the reactive stages of divorce and familiar with the inherent legal, custodial, financial, and social problems of the process. However, the proceedings of therapy are determined, as always, by the patient's characterological methods of coping and reacting, although these are now complicated by the process of mourning for the relationship and by the ever-shifting life situations involved.

Therapy moves beyond crisis intervention into a more thorough examination of underlying conflicts and lifelong patterns of interrelating, and a restructuring of these so that new patterns can emerge toward a healthier intrapsychic future.

Thus traditional models of psychodynamic psychotherapy must be adapted to the unusual set of circumstances. Initially, the person's history must be explored to reveal how earlier crises were handled, especially those involving narcissistic injury. Childhood and family ties and relationships must be explored. Prior identity formation, its foundations and development, must be clarified. The person's concept of marriage and marital roles must be discussed, as well as the evolution of the courtship and marriage and marital breakdown. Ties to friends must be analyzed, and usual ways of handling stress explored.

While all of these are becoming clear to the patient, ongoing realistic concerns intervene constantly. It is important to maintain a balance between support and reassurance, during particular crises over these events and during the process of psychotherapy. Often a session can be taken up by a pressing problem concerning legal or financial matters, but this can be used in the service of insight, as the therapist guides the patient toward an understanding of emotions and reactions in this event as examples of characteristic behavior. Low self-esteem can be bolstered by learning and practicing assertiveness techniques and by recognition of appropriate responses and functioning.

The therapist may encourage the patient to find community resource and support groups as necessary. This can be a beginning toward the establishment of new friendships to replace those lost with the marriage. For example, the patient may benefit from joining a group of other single parents or require direction in finding educational assistance for a child, or a religious counselor. The patient may need to be referred to employment agencies, educational facilities, or social assistance workers. The therapeutic process must not become sidetracked by these issues, but must incorporate them. At the same time, the patient is usually lonely and dependent. Therapy must deal openly with these emotions, and transference issues need to be dealt with thoroughly.

Feelings of failure must be addressed. Many women have been socialized to believe that if they are nice and good, they will be rewarded with love and acceptance. Divorce means that they have failed to be nice and good and thus deserve to be punished with rejection. This type of childhood primary thinking often conflicts with the adult reasoning that remains in control of the emotions and thus of self-esteem. She may then howl out her hurt and rage like a small child. This process takes many sessions to work through. The therapist who ignores this socialization aspect will too quickly label the patient as having a borderline personality disorder at this stage of therapy, especially if the rage progresses to self-abuse.

Instead, her reactions must be analyzed in terms of injured self-esteem, loss of feelings of personal mastery and control, and disappointment in her inability to fulfill her dream of "forever after" for the marriage. She is learning to change her self-concept, not only from the values she introjected in childhood from parents and others, but also from those she absorbed through the intricacies of the social and marital expectations of her as an adult woman. She is probably also encountering a variety of reactions to her changed status to a divorced woman and the societal stereotypes that still exist, for example, dealing with bank managers who refuse her loans, credit, or an overdraft because she is husbandless or learning how to reject unwanted sexual overtures from males ranging from relatives to repairmen. In short, she may be dealing with situations foreign to her as a "protected wife." Her identity therefore is being assaulted on all fronts.

Men also react to separation and divorce in ways determined by the sociocultural meaning of being a husband and in a marriage (see Chapter 3). The therapist has to be sensitive to the differing requirements of marriage between men and women and differing needs for intimacy, as discussed earlier in this chapter. Applying the same theories of interpersonal growth to both will result in a negative therapeutic experience.

Anger emerges in numerous and diverse ways, again often in ways characteristic throughout the person's life. A divorcing woman may behave unreasonably and irrationally only when communicating with her former spouse. She wonders why he can still anger and hurt her. Here his usual ways of interacting with her and with others must be examined. Gradually she learns to predict his behavior and responses to her and to be prepared to handle them. She begins to understand that her own personal growth is not reflected in a parallel change in him and that she cannot expect him to live up to her continuing hopes. At times, she idealizes the marriage and longs for its resumption while recognizing the impossibility of this. The positive aspects of the relationship can and should be acknowledged as well as the regret at their loss. The loss of the family unit needs discussion also and is particularly important to the noncustodial parent, many of whom will feel they have lost everything.

As therapy continues, the patient reports that she has had an increasing number of happy days, is enjoying her own company more, and is restructuring her life. Insights are being used, and personal growth is obvious. Once an equilibrium is established, therapy begins to conclude. Some new crises are weathered in new ways and the old patterns appear less frequently and more controllably.

The healing process continues for several years after a divorce. Ties between former spouses are difficult to dissolve, especially if they must interact because of their children. Psychotherapy helps the patient not only to complete the mourning and separation, but also to appropriately assess and accept responsibility for his or her contribution to the end of the marriage, rather than continuing on with blame and rage.

Divorce, though wrenching intrapsychically, can be the stimulus for personal growth and continuing development. With a firmer self-concept and greater self-esteem, no longer needing to fight old battles, the person is free to form a new relationship.

References

1. Holmes TR, Rahe RH: The Social Readjustment Rating Scale. J Psychosom Med 2:213-218, 1967

2. Paykel ES, Prusoff BA, Uhlenhuth EH: Scaling of life events. Arch Gen Psychiatry 25:340-347, 1971
3. National Center for Health Statistics: Births, marriages, divorce, and deaths for January, 1986. Monthly Vital Statistics Report (DHHS publication no. [PHS] 86-1120), April 21, 1986
4. Ministry of Justice: Divorce in Canada: Proposals for Change. Ottawa, Department of Supply and Services, 1984
5. Hunt MM: Alone, alone, all, all alone, in Loneliness: The Experience of Emotional and Social Isolation. Edited by Weiss RS. Cambridge, The MIT Press, 1973
6. Jacobson GF: The multiple crises of marital separation and divorce, in Seminars in Psychiatry. Edited by Greenblatt M. New York, Grune and Stratton, 1983
7. Erikson E: Identity: Youth and Crisis. New York, W.W. Norton, 1968
8. Gilligan C: In a Different Voice. Cambridge, MA, Harvard University Press, 1982
9. Greatrex TES: Separation and divorce: crisis and development, in Treatment Interventions in Human Sexuality. Edited by Nadelson CC, Marcotte DB. New York, Plenum Press, 1983
10. Kaslow FW: Stages of divorce: a psychological perspective. Villanova Law Review 25:718-751, 1979/80
11. Spira L: The experience of divorce for the psychotherapy patient—a developmental perspective. Clinical Social Work Journal 9:258-270, 1981